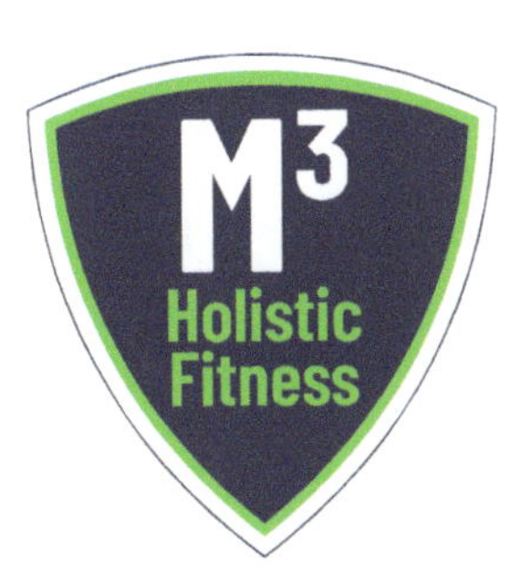

RISE AND ALIGN

90-DAY HOLISTIC FITNESS JOURNAL

M3 Holistic Fitness Journal

ISBN Paperback: 979-8-9900832-2-6
ISBN eBook: 979-8-9900832-3-3

First Edition
Version 12.2024 | December 2024
Series: M3 Holistic Fitness/ M3 Holistic Fitness series

Published by: M3 Holistic Media LLC
Palm Springs, California
Email: M3HolisticMedia@gmail.com

Editor: Book Your Brand LLC | David Strauss

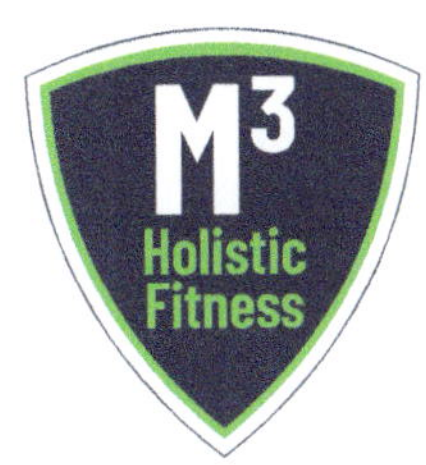

Welcome to Your 90-Day M3 Fitness Journal
Our Journey Together

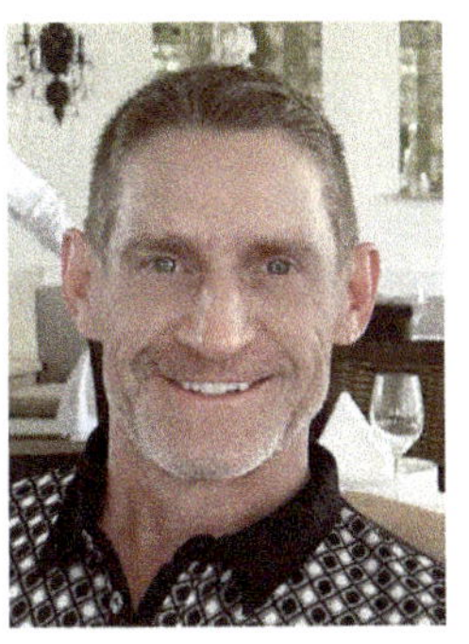

Hey there! I'm Dirk Schultz, and I'm excited you've decided to embark on this 90-day journey with me using the M3 Method. This journal will be your companion through the next three months, guiding you to integrate the pillars of Mindset, Movement, and Meals into your life.

I've spent years exploring fitness and wellness, and the M3 Method was born from the realization that true health isn't just about physical strength—it's about finding harmony between your mind, body, and spirit. Over the next 90 days, this journal will help you track your progress, reflect on your habits, and stay motivated as you work toward a more energized and fulfilling life.

The M3 Method stands for Mindset, Movement, and Meals—three pillars that I believe are essential for creating a fulfilling and balanced life.

Mindset: Set intentions, practice positive thinking, and stay mentally strong.

Movement: Explore and track a variety of activities that fit your lifestyle.

Meals: Plan and reflect on balanced, nourishing meals that support overall well-being.

This journal is about creating a life that feels amazing—inside and out. Whether you want to improve your energy, health, or find more joy, the M3 Method will guide you. Let's make the next 90 days count!

— Dirk Schultz

The Transformative Power of the M3 Method: A Holistic Approach to a Happier, Healthier You

The M3 Method is built on three pillars—Mindset, Movement, and Meals—to help you live a life that feels as good as it looks. By embracing these elements, you're setting yourself up for a life that's not just healthier but richer in every sense. Here's how the M3 Method can transform you:

---

1. Holistic Well-Being

The M3 Method nurtures your mind, body, and spirit, creating a balanced life. This integration fosters mental sharpness, emotional resilience, and physical health, helping you handle challenges with ease.

2. Increased Energy and Vitality

By fueling your body with nutritious meals, regular movement, and a positive mindset, you'll experience a noticeable boost in energy. You'll wake up feeling refreshed and ready for the day.

3. Enhanced Mental Clarity and Focus

Mindfulness, physical activity, and balanced nutrition improve focus, reduce mental fog, and sharpen your memory, helping you stay on track with your goals.

4. Emotional Resilience

A strong mindset and stress-reducing activities build emotional stability. By maintaining a positive outlook and nourishing your body, you become more resilient to life's ups and downs.

5. Improved Physical Health

Movement and nutrition go beyond basics in the M3 Method—they're about finding joy in activities you enjoy and meals that satisfy. This makes it easier to stick to healthy habits, leading to better strength, flexibility, and endurance.

6. Stronger Relationships

As you enhance your mental and emotional health, you'll find your relationships becoming more fulfilling and supportive. The M3 Method encourages self-awareness and emotional intelligence, key to stronger connections.

7. Purpose and Fulfillment

When your daily actions align with your values, your sense of purpose deepens. The M3 Method helps you live intentionally, bringing fulfillment and meaning to your life.

8. Sustainable Lifestyle Changes

Instead of quick fixes, the M3 Method promotes gradual, lasting changes that become a natural part of your life. This sustainability ensures long-term health and happiness.

9. Increased Longevity and Quality of Life

By taking care of your mind, body, and spirit, you not only add years to your life but enhance the quality of those years. The M3 Method helps you age with vitality, staying active and engaged for years to come.

10. A Life of Joy and Ease

When your mind is clear, body strong, and spirit uplifted, life flows with more joy and ease. The M3 Method offers a path to a life that feels as good as it looks.

Mindset: The Foundation of Growth

The M3 Method encourages cultivating a positive, growth-oriented mindset. This involves self-awareness, setting daily intentions, building resilience, and practicing positive affirmations. With the right mindset, you'll be better equipped to overcome challenges and stay focused on your goals.

Movement: Joy in Staying Active

Movement should feel good, not like a chore. The M3 Method encourages finding activities that you enjoy, whether that's yoga, dancing, or walking. It's about consistent, sustainable movement that makes you feel energized and connected to your body.

Meals: Nourishing Body, Mind, and Soul

The M3 Method emphasizes mindful, balanced eating—real, whole foods that nourish your body. It's not about restrictive diets but about enjoying meals that make you feel your best. Mindful eating also means paying attention to how and what you eat, listening to your body's needs.

Bringing It All Together

Mindset, Movement, and Meals work in harmony to create lasting change. Small, sustainable shifts lead to big results over time, whether you're looking to boost your energy, improve health, or experience more joy in daily life. The M3 Method is a commitment to yourself—a path to living a balanced, healthy, and fulfilling life.

Are you ready to embrace the transformative power of the M3 Method? Let's make it a reality, one step at a time.

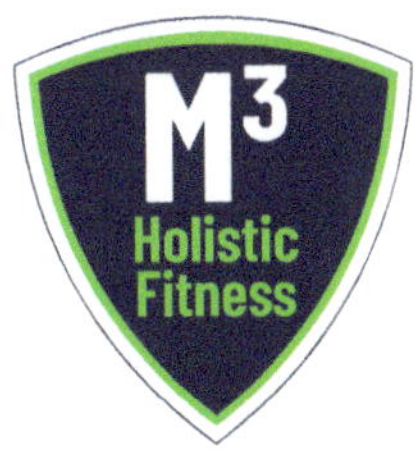

Welcome to a journey that's about to redefine your approach to health, vitality, and personal fulfillment!

As you turn each page of this M3 Method Journal, prepare to embark on an adventure of personal transformation—a complete reset of how you think about wellness, focusing on the **M3 Method: Mindset, Movement, Meals.**

This isn't just about physical fitness; it's about embracing a lifestyle that harmonizes your mental, emotional, and spiritual well-being with your physical health. Get ready to dive into a method that's tailored just for you, bringing clarity, energy, and joy into every aspect of your life.

Whether you're looking to revitalize your body, rejuvenate your mind, or realign your life goals, the M3 Method is your comprehensive guide. It's designed to spark a deep transformation that goes beyond the surface, touching every part of your existence.

With practical tools, insightful prompts, and supportive advice, this journal is more than just a notebook—it's a daily companion on your path to becoming the most vibrant version of yourself.

The M3 Way

The M3 Method is more than a wellness program; it's a holistic blueprint for achieving both physical fitness and emotional, mental, and spiritual well-being. This approach encourages you to live consciously, immersing yourself fully in each moment while being mindful of what you put in your mind and body.

The M3 Method isn't just helpful—it's transformational. It brings daily structure and lifestyle choices into focus, which you can either tackle solo or make it a group effort within your community. The M3 Method is a much-needed path to peace of mind. The M3 Method steps up as your go-to roadmap, enhancing your quality of life as you journey through creating the life you want.

The dynamic interplay among the M3 Method's three core pillars—Mindset, Movement, and Meals—is vividly illustrated in the following diagram:

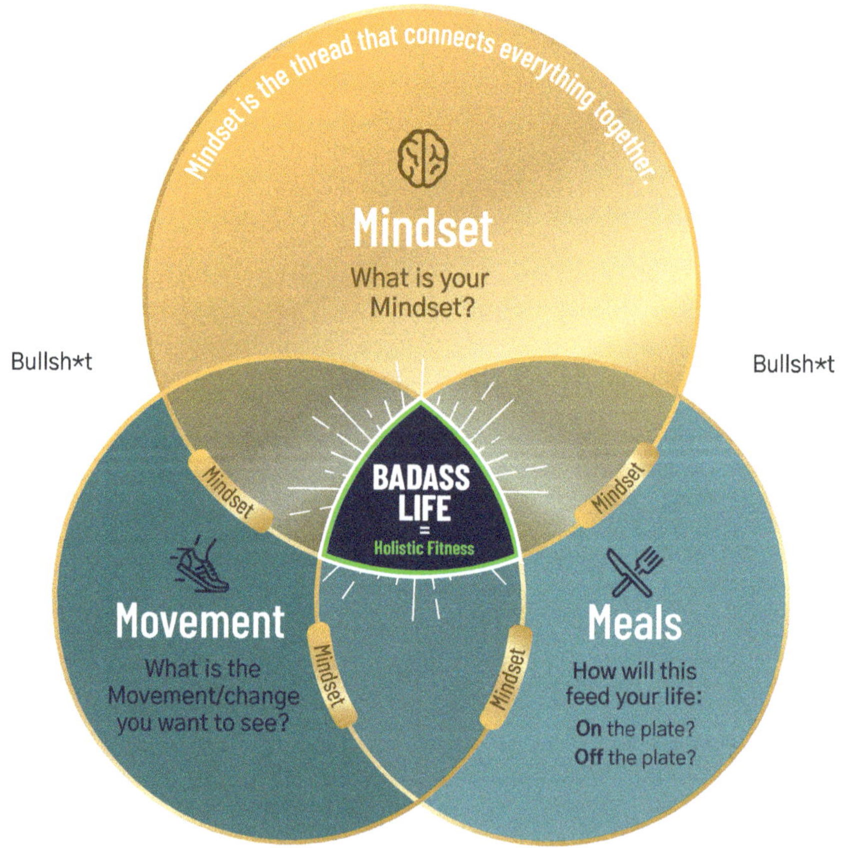

Each element is a standalone powerhouse for your well-being, but their synergy propels your wellness to the next level. This cooperative interaction sets the stage for a holistic transformation that transcends a basic health plan; it's a full-scale lifestyle overhaul that seamlessly integrates physical, mental, and spiritual aspects of well-being.

Starting your journey with the M3 Method is a long-term commitment built upon a focus that thrives on continual growth. As you traverse the path to holistic health, you'll learn to cherish each moment and celebrate every achievement, big or small.

Remember, the road to ultimate wellness isn't just a straight shot or a dull stroll; it's a rollercoaster ride full of scenic routes, peaks, valleys, and eye-popping vistas. The M3 Method is your co-pilot on this thrilling journey, serving as your all-in-one toolkit for life enhancement. It arms you with a rock-solid Mindset to conquer challenges, revs you up with Movement that energizes every fiber of your being, and satisfies your soul with Meals that go beyond mere calories. Within this dynamic framework, each step you take isn't just incremental progress; it's a turbo boost that elevates your entire quality of life. So, buckle up, and let's make this ride an exhilarating one!

The M3 Rise and Align Journal

The M3 Journal is the ultimate playbook where you sketch, plan, and celebrate your journey to becoming the most BADASS version of yourself!

It isn't just a notebook; it's the canvas where you paint the portrait of your most BADASS self. This transformative journal fuses everything we've talked about—the M3 Method and the BADASS lifestyle—into a daily practice that you can literally hold in your hands. Picture it as your life's roadmap, brimming with the colors of Mindset, Movement, and Meals.

Mindset gets its rightful spotlight in this journal. You'll find sections dedicated to your goals, affirmations, and reflections. This is your safe space to jot down the thoughts that uplift you and confront those that hold you back. It's where your mental game gets fine-tuned, helping you embody that bursting enthusiasm and empowering attitude we talked about.

Movement isn't just penciled in—it's highlighted, circled, and underlined. Your M3 Journal comes with pages that encourage you to log your physical activities, whether it's hitting the gym, doing yoga, or going for a nature hike. Here, you channel your determination to succeed and build up the stamina to go the distance. Each entry becomes a badge of honor, showcasing your unwavering commitment to staying active and fierce.

Then there's **Meals**, and we're talking about nourishment in its broadest sense. In this part of the journal, you capture everything that fuels you. From the food you eat to your relationships, career, physical activity, and creativity, just to name a few, that you nurture; you'll have designated space to reflect on the elements that enrich your life. This is where you dig deep into the self–belief that grounds you and the ambition that fuels your dreams.

Beyond the triple M's, your M3 Journal will have prompts that foster continuous self-development. It's the nudge you need to engage in intellectual nourishment and emotional growth, tying back into the BADASS qualities you aim to embody.

So, if you're ready to take your life from good to epic, the M3 Journal is your partner in crime. With it, you're not just jotting down words; you're scripting the compelling narrative of your BADASS journey. Consider this journal your daily dose of M3 goodness, an intimate dialogue with yourself that guides, celebrates, and propels you into a life that's as enriching as it is exhilarating.

Grab that pen, my friend. Your BADASS LIFE is waiting to be written.

Creating the Life You Want Game Plan

M3 Circle of Life

As your eyes glide over the M3 Circle of Life diagram below, you'll notice it's sliced into three delicious pie sections: Mindset, Movement, and Meals. Each slice is jam-packed with specifics to dive into.

Imagine this: a life where your Mindset, Movement, and Meals seamlessly blend together, each one amplifying the others. It's more than just a healthy lifestyle; it's a state of effortless flow enriched with purpose and intention. In this reality, your mental clarity influences your physical activity, nourishing your dietary choices. It's a harmonious cycle where every element is dialed in, and the result is a version of you optimized for joy, wellness, and meaningful connections. As you journey through this journal, we will delve into the unique sub-elements that form each of the three M3 pillars. This will equip you with a comprehensive toolbox for crafting a life that's both good and extraordinary.

Non-Negotiables

A non-negotiable is a sacred commitment you make with yourself—a daily habit or action that aligns you with the life you want to create. It's a promise that says, "No matter what, I will show up for myself today." Whether it's for your health, fitness, finances, relationships, or community, these non-negotiables are the foundation of lasting change. In the M3 Method, non-negotiables form the bedrock of your journey, providing structure and accountability as you consistently take small, intentional actions toward your goals. When you honor your non-negotiables, you honor your potential, setting a powerful standard for how you live, grow, and thrive within the M3 Method. Below are some examples of non-negotiable under each of the M3 pillars, use some of these or let them inspire you to come up with your own.

DAY / HABIT	Journaling	Balanced Nutrition	Stretching Routine	Mindful Reflection	Step Count Goal	Strength Training	Meal Planning
1	✓	✓	✓	✓	✓	✓	✓
2	✓	✓	✓	✓	✓		✓
3	✓	✓	✓	✓	✓	✓	✓
4	✓	✓	✓	✓	✓		✓
5	✓	✓	✓	✓	✓		✓
6	✓	✓	✓	✓	✓		✓
7	✓	✓	✓	✓	✓	✓	✓
8	✓	✓	✓	✓	✓		✓
9	✓	✓	✓	✓	✓		✓
10	✓	✓	✓	✓	✓	✓	✓
11	✓	✓	✓	✓	✓		✓
12	✓	✓	✓	✓	✓	✓	✓
13	✓	✓	✓	✓	✓	✓	✓
14	✓	✓	✓	✓	✓		✓

MINDSET NON-NEGOTIABLES

1. Daily Gratitude Practice

Every morning, I will write down three things I am grateful for to start my day with a positive and abundant mindset.

2. Mindful Reflection

I will take 10 minutes each evening to reflect on the day's successes and challenges, reinforcing a growth mindset.

3. Affirmation Practice

Every day, I will say or write my personal affirmations to reprogram my subconscious toward my goals.

4. Visualization

I will dedicate 5 minutes daily to visualize the outcome I desire, connecting emotionally to my future success.

5. Journaling

Every morning, I will write down three things I am grateful for to start my day with a positive and abundant mindset.

MOVEMENT NON-NEGOTIABLES

1. Daily Movement

I will engage in at least 30 minutes of intentional movement, whether through walking, yoga, or exercise, to keep my body active.

2. Stretching Routine

I will take 10 minutes every morning to stretch my body, enhancing flexibility and preparing for the day ahead.

3. Step Count Goal

I will aim for a daily step goal (e.g., 10,000 steps) to ensure I stay physically active throughout the day.

4. Weekly Strength Training

I will include strength training in my routine at least 3 times per week to build and maintain muscle health.

5. Rest and Recovery

I will prioritize 7–8 hours of quality sleep each night to support recovery and overall well-being.

MEALS NON-NEGOTIABLES

1. Mindful Eating

I will eat each meal mindfully, savoring the flavors, and chewing slowly to fully enjoy and properly digest my food.

2. Hydration

I will drink at least 8 glasses of water daily to stay hydrated and support my body's natural functions.

3. Balanced Nutrition

Every meal will include a balance of protein, healthy fats, and vegetables to nourish my body and maintain energy levels.

4. Meal Planning

I will plan my meals for the week in advance to ensure I make healthy choices and avoid impulsive eating.

5. No Processed Sugar

I will avoid processed sugars in my meals to maintain consistent energy and promote long-term health..

These non-negotiables reflect a holistic commitment to personal growth, physical health, and balanced living, all while staying aligned with the M3 Method's Mindset, Movement, Meals philosophy.

Make it Happen This Week

Use this for recording and monitoring your weekly actions and tasks in the areas of Mindset, Movement and Meals.

You can also use this section to record your daily activities and progress with your Monthly Non-Negotiables.

At the end of each day, this will help you review your accomplishments and reflect on areas for growth.

	MINDSET	MOVEMENT	MEALS ✔ ON THE PLATE	✔ OFF THE PLATE
MON	Reviewed Wellness vision for the week 10 min meditation	Yoga Class @ 6:00pm	Chicken Breast Side Salad Green Beans	Volunteer 1hr at the animal shelter
TUES	Listen to Podcast on the drive to work	50 min Strength training	Oatmeal w/berries Veggie burger Sweet potato fries	50 min phone call w/ best friends
WEDS	Start the day w/gratitude	Use the stairs at work 45 min brisk walk after work	Baked Salmon w/lemon and a salad	Meet friends for game night
THURS	Attending online M3 Mastermind 5:30pm	50 min Strength training 10 min stretch	Turkey Burger w/broccoli slaw	Movie Night
FRI	Repeat morning affirmation	Brisk walk through the neighbourhood	Eggplant parmesan + salad	Happy Hour w/friends

Taking a holistic approach to your wellness

The Morning Rise and Align

Remember, the most effective morning ritual is the one that resonates with you and complements your lifestyle. Be flexible and open to adjustments as you discover what practices serve you best. Your ritual may evolve with you, reflecting changes in your schedule, priorities, or wellness goals. Also, don't pressure yourself to create an elaborate morning ritual overnight. Start small, perhaps with just one or two practices, and gradually incorporate more elements. Consistency, not complexity, is the key to a successful morning ritual. A morning ritual is not merely a sequence of tasks but a harmonious symphony of habits that sing to the rhythm of your well-being. By making the choice to rise and align each morning, you're not only investing in your health and fitness but also in your growth as a person. Embrace the beauty of a purposeful morning and witness the profound impact it has on the trajectory of your day and, ultimately, your life.

Record your hours of sleep, energy level, mood, and hydration.

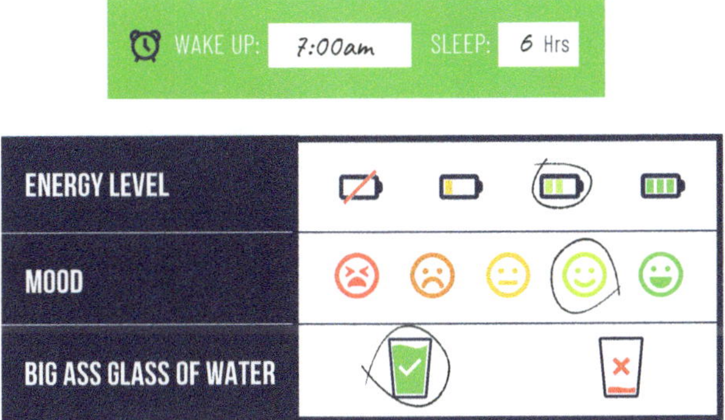

What Am I Grateful For?

Cultivate Gratitude

Beginning your day with a sense of gratitude can elevate your mood and broaden your perspective. A daily gratitude practice, such as writing down three things you're thankful for, can shift your focus from what's lacking in your life to what is abundant.

I AM GRATEFUL FOR:

Daily Intention

Set Intention Goals

Before the day sweeps you up in its ebb and flow, take a moment to outline your objectives. What do you want to achieve today? Setting clear, achievable goals can channel your energy towards meaningful action. It also provides a sense of accomplishment when you tick off completed tasks.

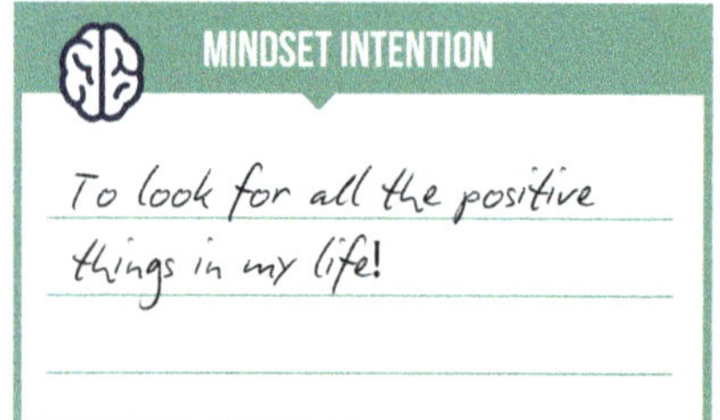

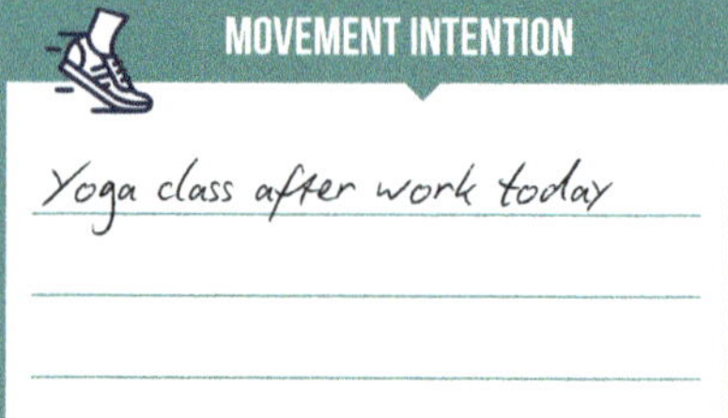

MEALS INTENTION

✔ **ON** THE PLATE

Turkey Burger   Broccoli   Salad
Frozen Yogurt

✔ **OFF** THE PLATE

Game Night with Friends

MINDFUL AFFIRMATION:

I joyfully accept wealth and prosperity into my life

Night Cap

Your evening nightcap is more than just a winding-down routine; it's an essential ritual that balances your day and prepares you for what's ahead. Spend a few quiet moments reflecting on the day's highs and lows, perhaps jotting them down in a journal. This practice not only helps you process emotions but also serves as a springboard for setting tomorrow's intentions.

Bed Time: Record the time you go to bed. This will help you create a consistent sleep routine.

Hydration: Record how many ounces of water you consumed during the day.

Our bodies are mostly water, a fluid medium that's essential for the smooth execution of countless biochemical reactions. From energy production and nutrient distribution to waste elimination, hydration is the silent facilitator of our overall health. Keep yourself well-hydrated, and you're not just satisfying thirst—you're fueling your metabolism, sharpening your mind, and optimizing nutrient delivery. It's vital to acknowledge that hydration needs aren't uniform—they vary based on factors like climate, activity level, age, and individual health conditions. But a general rule of thumb is around 90–126 ounces daily.

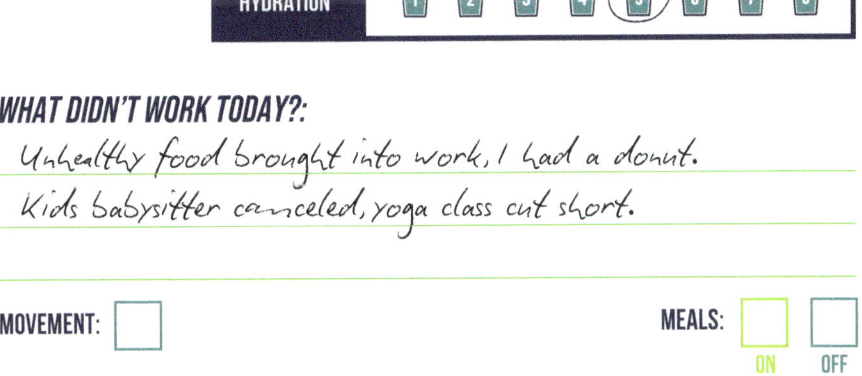

WHAT DIDN'T WORK TODAY?:

Unhealthy food brought into work, I had a donut.

Kids babysitter canceled, yoga class cut short.

MOVEMENT: ☐

MEALS: ☐ ☐
ON   OFF

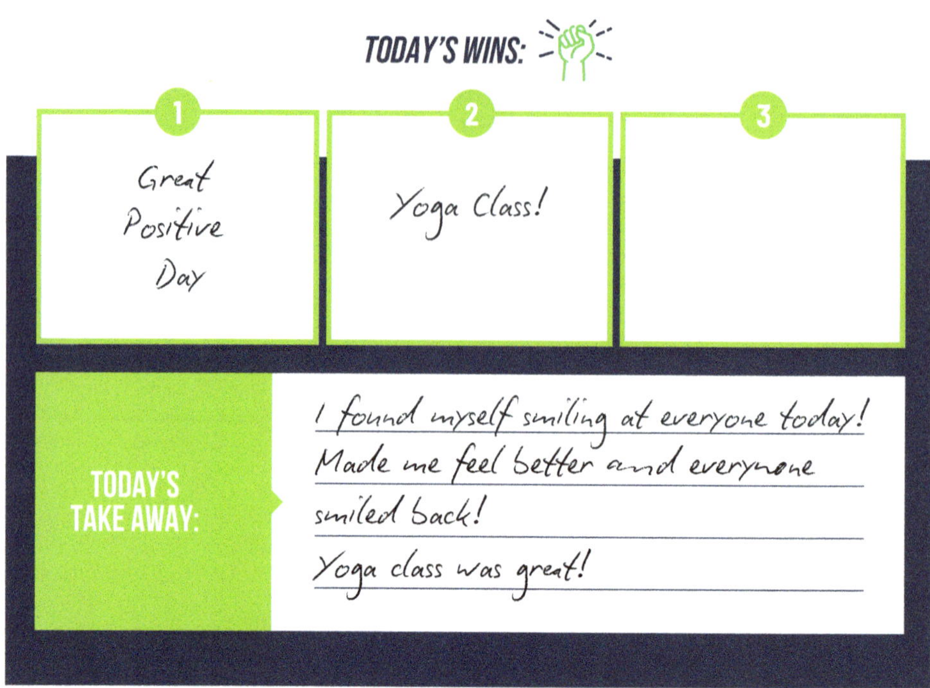

FOOD FOR THOUGHT FOR THE DAY:

Tomorrow is another chance to start over!
Tomorrow will even be better than today!

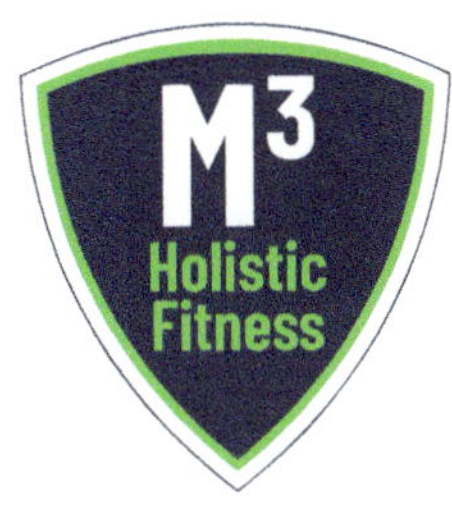

The M3 Four Agreements

Mindset Agreement: I agree and commit to developing a growth mindset, envisioning what I want for my life, and embracing a "can do" attitude. I will prioritize my well-being, celebrate the wisdom gained from my experiences, and live authentically, driven by my "why."

Movement Agreement: I agree and commit to moving with intention, recognizing the importance of both physical and mental health. I will engage in forms of movement that reflect my life's journey, expressing my authentic self through activities that nourish my body and soul.

Meals Agreement: I agree and commit to nourishing both my body and spirit through mindful eating and embracing the connection between food, memory, and identity. I will also nurture my life off the plate, feeding areas like relationships, creativity, and spirituality to create balance and fulfillment.

Tribe Agreement: I agree and commit to embracing my community and actively nurturing connections with those who resonate with my journey. I will be a source of support and lean on my tribe when needed, knowing that together we thrive and elevate our holistic well-being.

This next 90 days is about me. I will take the action needed to step into the next best version of myself.

Signature: _______________________   Date: _______________

ACTION

A | **Align with your vision:** Make your vision a daily habit. Own it, visualize it, feel it, and embody it. Visualize your goals and success regularly to stay focused and motivated on your journey.

C | **Conquer your fears:** Don't let fear hold you back. Face your fears head–on, identify where they come from, and change your relationship with them. As the saying goes, "Face your fears and do it anyway." Remember that fear and excitement originate from the same place, so flip the script and replace fear with excitement.

T | **Team up with supportive people:** Share your goals with your family, friends, mentors, and those who genuinely support and hold you accountable. These are the folks who uplift you and celebrate your journey and achievements with true enthusiasm.

I | **Invest in yourself:** Dedicate your time, money, and energy to propel yourself forward and make your vision a reality. Prioritize self–improvement, education, and self–care to lay a solid foundation for your success.

O | **Organize your plan:** Put your plan down in detail, breaking it into manageable steps. Review it daily to ensure you stay on track and be ready to adapt when necessary.

N | **Navigate your next best move and seize the moment:**
Choose one or two actions to commit to and take them now. Remember that any forward movement, regardless of its size, generates momentum, and each step matters. You can't adjust your course if you're standing still, so embrace the present and get started now! Enjoy the journey, learn from your experiences, and always remember that the time to act is right now. Have fun along the way!

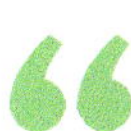

To accomplish great things we must not only act, but also dream; not only plan, but also believe.

-Anatole France

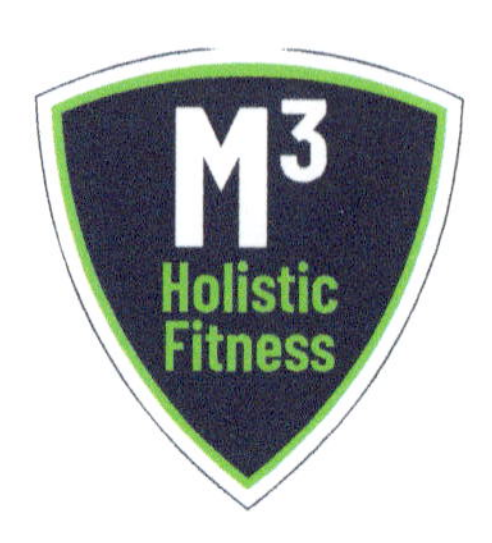

WEEK 1

90-DAY HOLISTIC FITNESS JOURNAL

M³ CIRCLE OF LIFE

WHAT DOES *YOUR* LIFE LOOK LIKE?

1. Place a dot in each category to indicate your level of satisfaction within each area. A dot at the **center of the circle to indicate dissatisfaction**, or towards the **outer edge to indicate satisfaction**. Most people fall somewhere in between. (see example)

2. Connect the dots to see your M₃ Circle of Life.

3. Identify imbalances. Determine where to spend more time and energy to create balance. **This will help you create a better balance for your best Badass Life.**

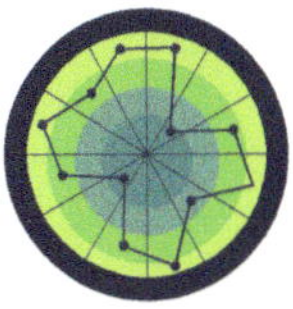

SATISFACTION

DISSATISFACTION

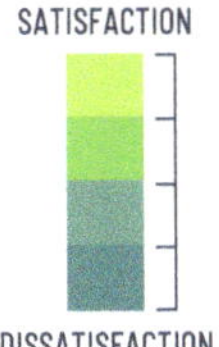

EXAMPLE

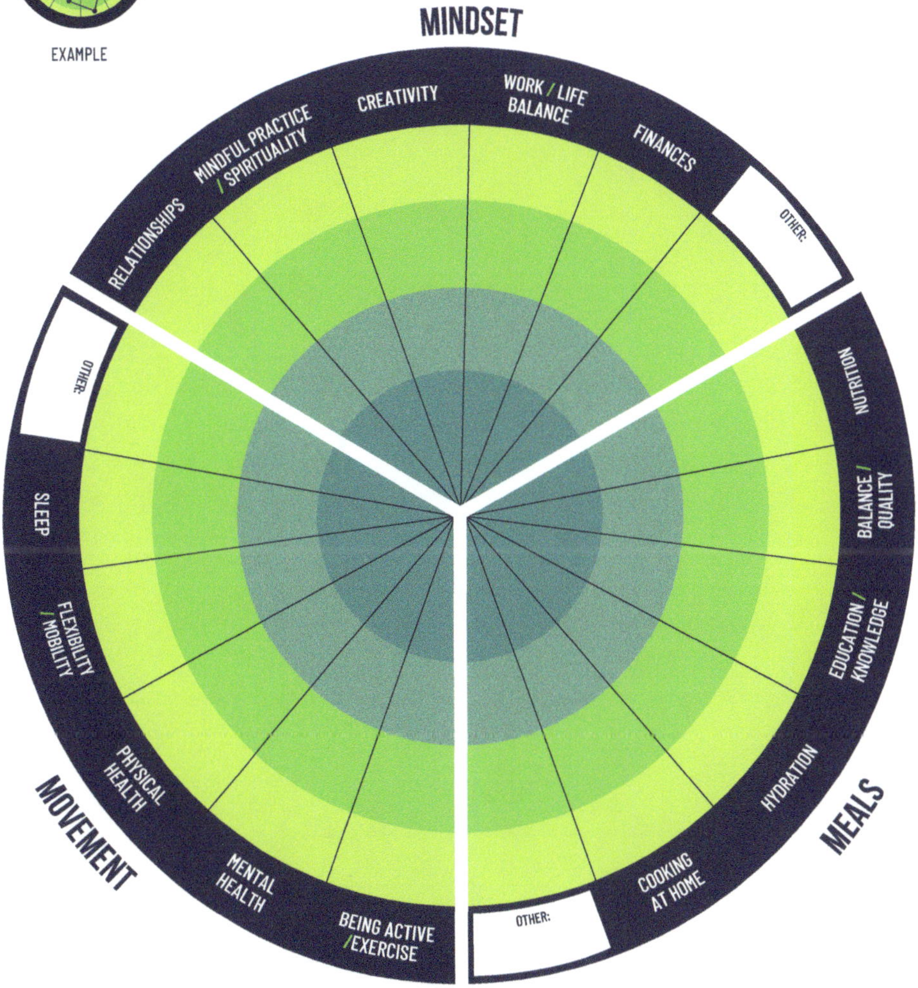

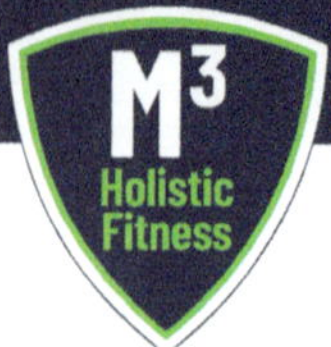

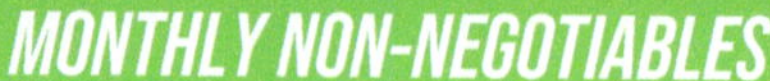

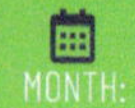

MONTH:

HABIT							

DAY							
1							
2							
3							
4							
5							
6							
7							
8							
9							
10							
11							
12							
13							
14							
15							
16							
17							
18							
19							
20							
21							
22							
23							
24							
25							
26							
27							
28							
29							
30							
31							
TOTAL							

M3 Holistic Fitness

MAKE IT HAPPEN THIS WEEK

WEEK OF: ___ / ___ / ___

	MINDSET	MOVEMENT	MEALS ON THE PLATE	 OFF THE PLATE
MON				
TUES				
WEDS				
THURS				
FRI				
SAT				
SUN				

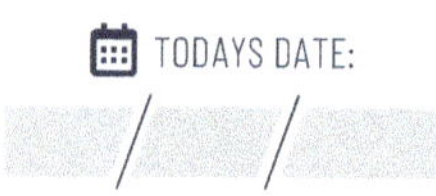

📅 TODAYS DATE: ____ / ____ / ____

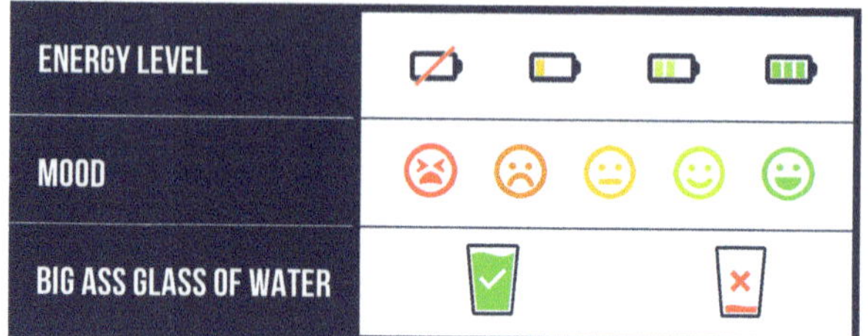

ENERGY LEVEL				
MOOD	😣	🙁	😐	🙂 😀
BIG ASS GLASS OF WATER	✓		✗	

I AM GRATEFUL FOR:

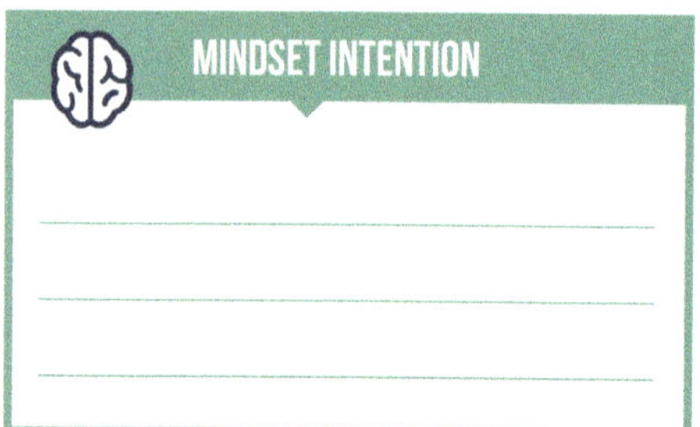

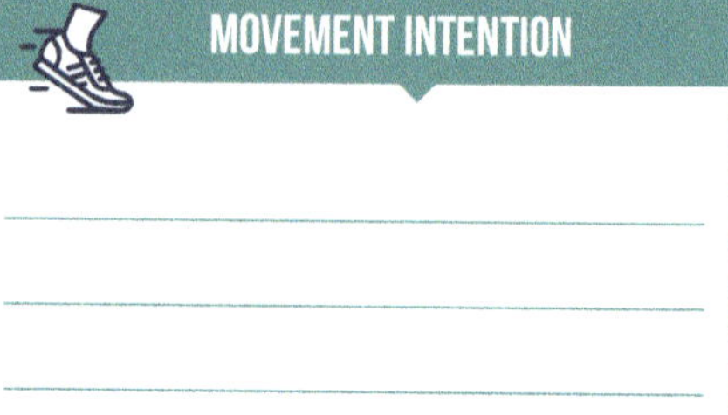

MINDFUL AFFIRMATION:

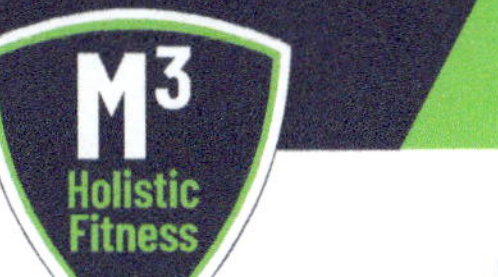

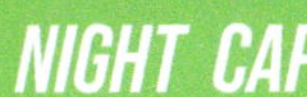

BEDTIME:

HYDRATION 1 2 3 4 5 6 7 8

WHAT DIDN'T WORK TODAY?:

MOVEMENT: ☐

MEALS: ☐ ON ☐ OFF

TODAY'S WINS:

1

2

3

TODAY'S TAKE AWAY:

FOOD FOR THOUGHT FOR THE DAY:

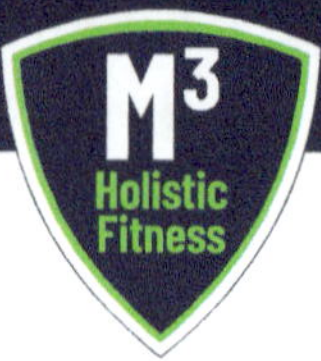

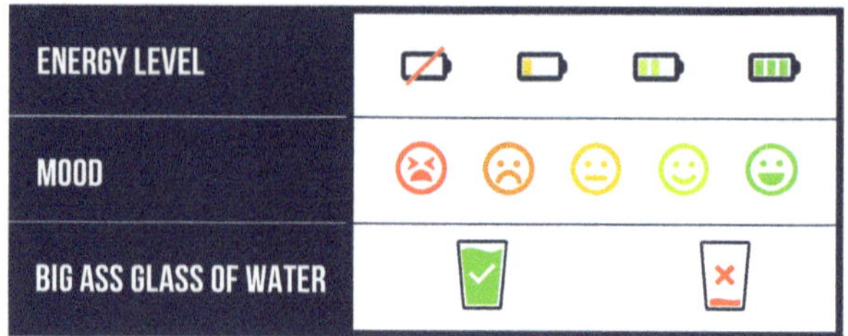

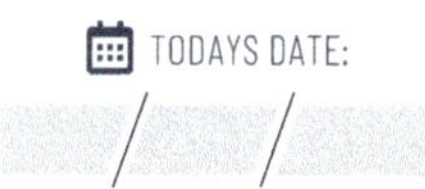

TODAYS DATE: _____ / _____ / _____

ENERGY LEVEL				
MOOD				
BIG ASS GLASS OF WATER				

I AM GRATEFUL FOR:

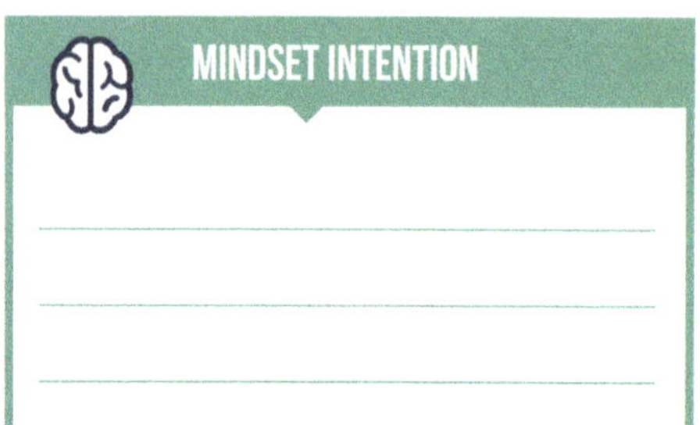

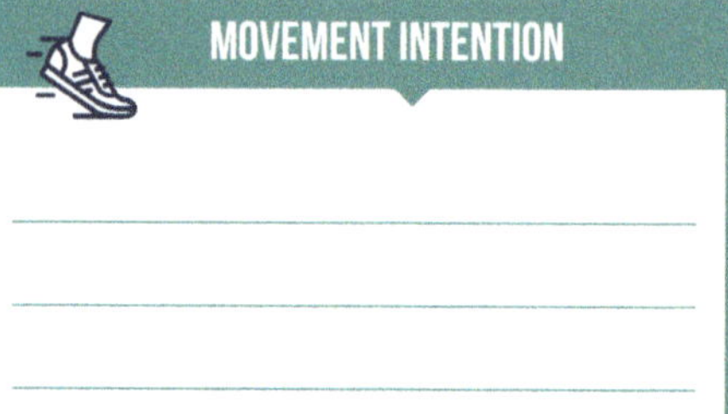

MINDFUL AFFIRMATION:

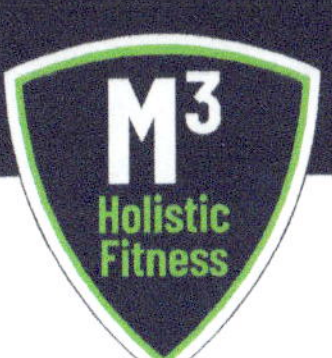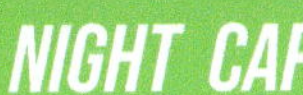# NIGHT CAP

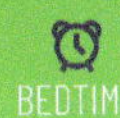 BEDTIME:

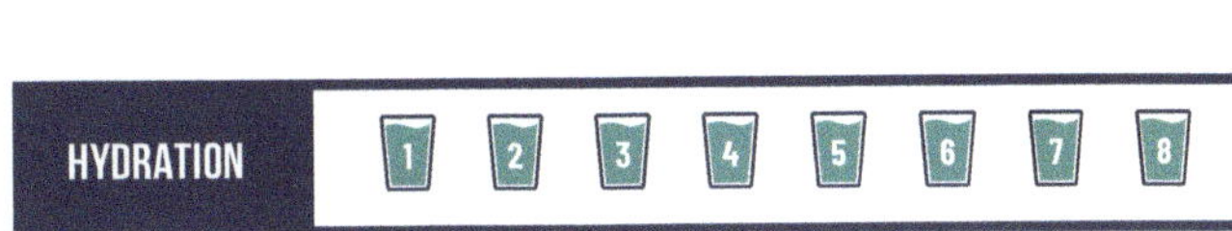

HYDRATION 1 2 3 4 5 6 7 8

WHAT DIDN'T WORK TODAY?:

MOVEMENT: ☐

MEALS: ☐ ON ☐ OFF

TODAY'S WINS:

1

2

3

TODAY'S TAKE AWAY:

FOOD FOR THOUGHT FOR THE DAY:

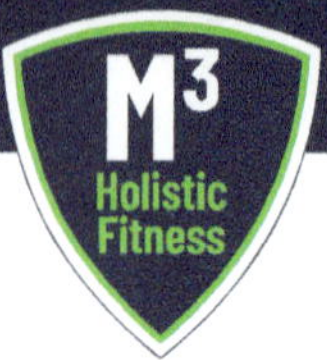

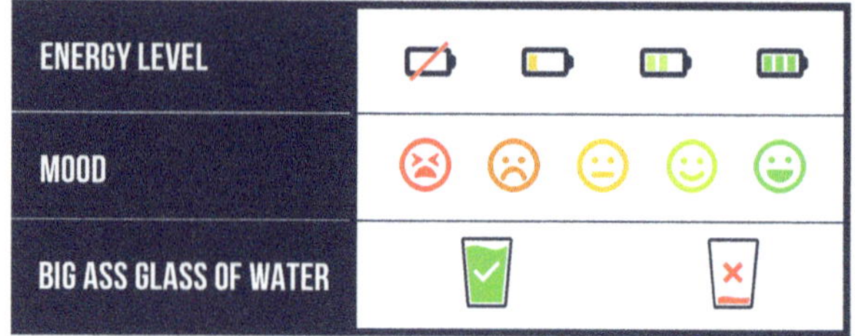

M³
Holistic
Fitness

TODAYS DATE:
_____ / _____ / _____

I AM GRATEFUL FOR:

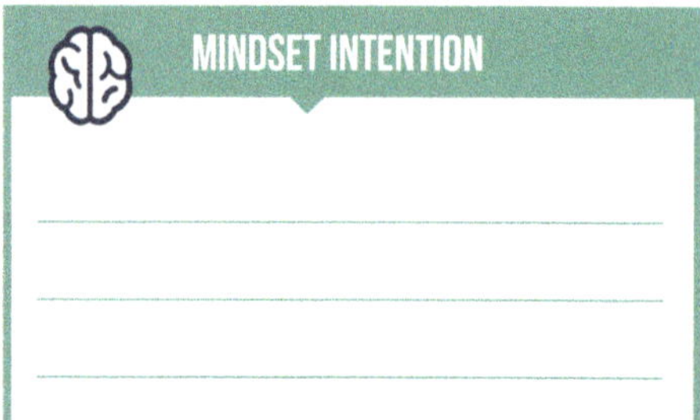

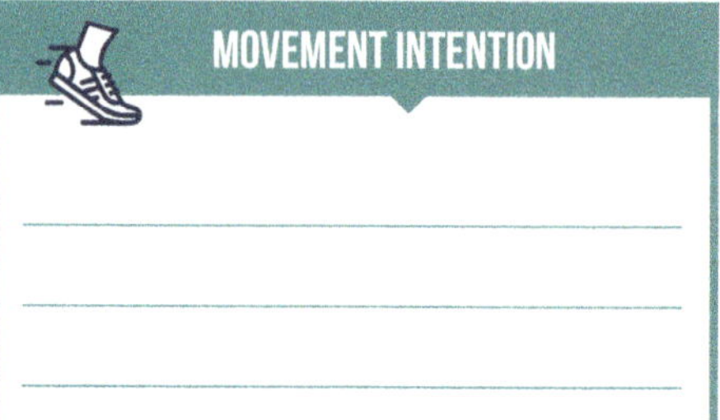

MINDFUL AFFIRMATION:

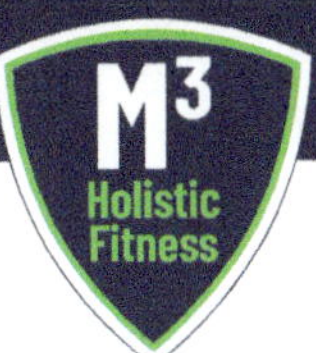

BEDTIME:

HYDRATION 1 2 3 4 5 6 7 8

WHAT DIDN'T WORK TODAY?:

MOVEMENT:

MEALS:
ON   OFF

TODAY'S WINS: 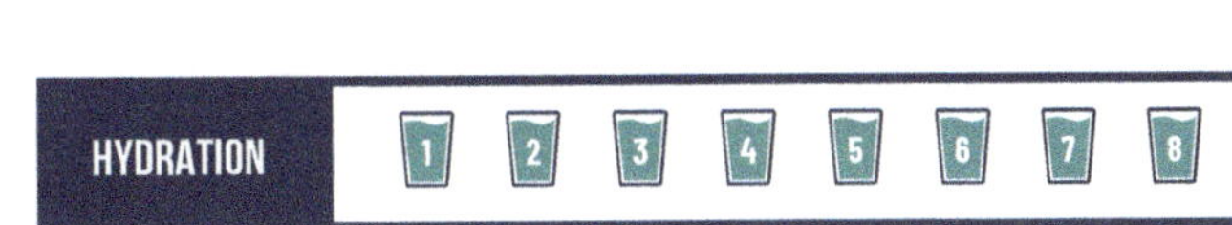

1

2

3

TODAY'S
TAKE AWAY:

FOOD FOR THOUGHT FOR THE DAY:

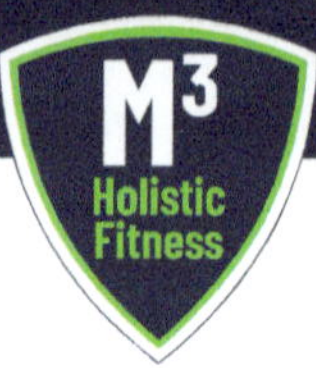

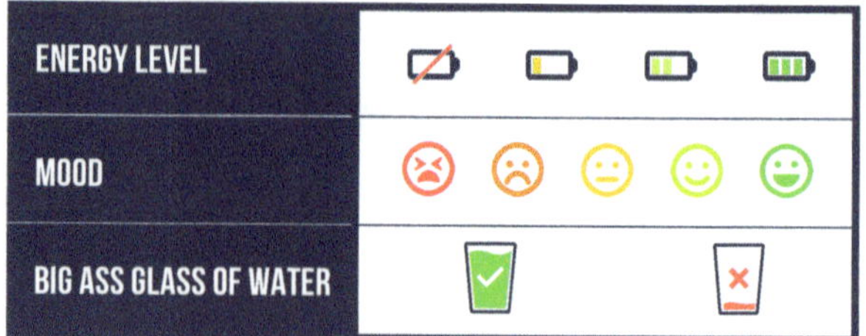

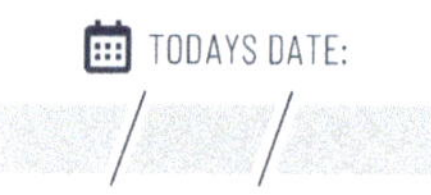

ENERGY LEVEL	
MOOD	
BIG ASS GLASS OF WATER	

I AM GRATEFUL FOR:

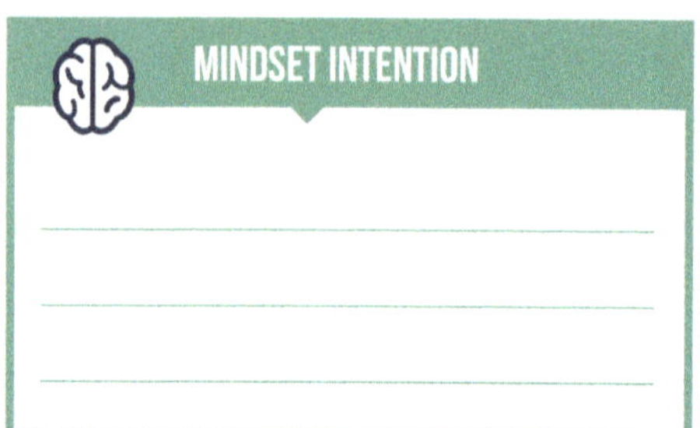

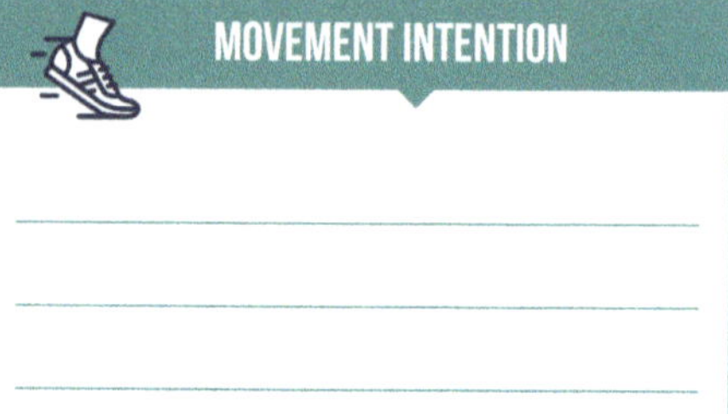

MINDFUL AFFIRMATION:

HYDRATION 1 2 3 4 5 6 7 8

WHAT DIDN'T WORK TODAY?:

MOVEMENT: ☐

MEALS: ☐ ON ☐ OFF

TODAY'S WINS: 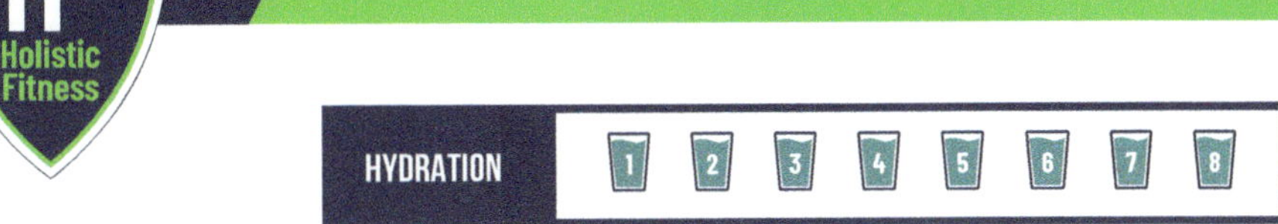

1

2

3

TODAY'S TAKE AWAY:

FOOD FOR THOUGHT FOR THE DAY:

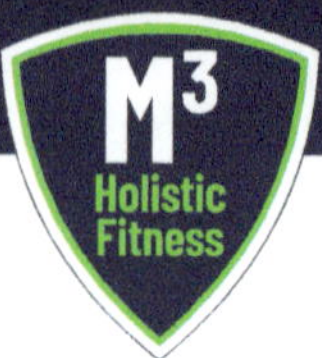

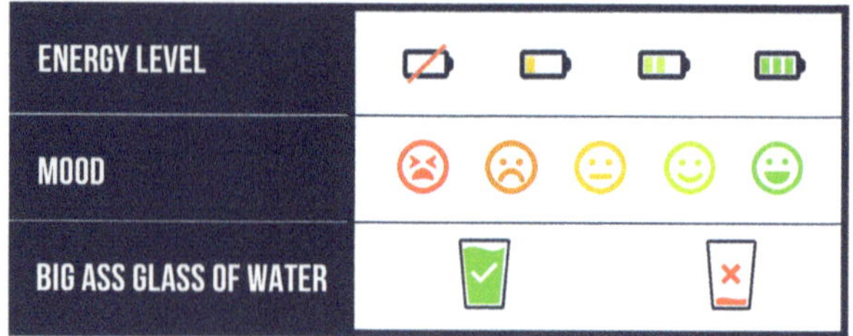

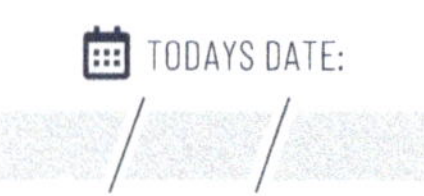

TODAYS DATE:

_____ / _____ / _____

ENERGY LEVEL				
MOOD				
BIG ASS GLASS OF WATER				

I AM GRATEFUL FOR:

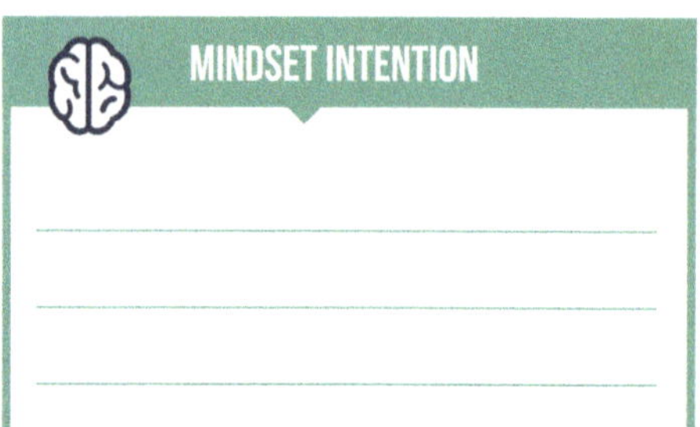

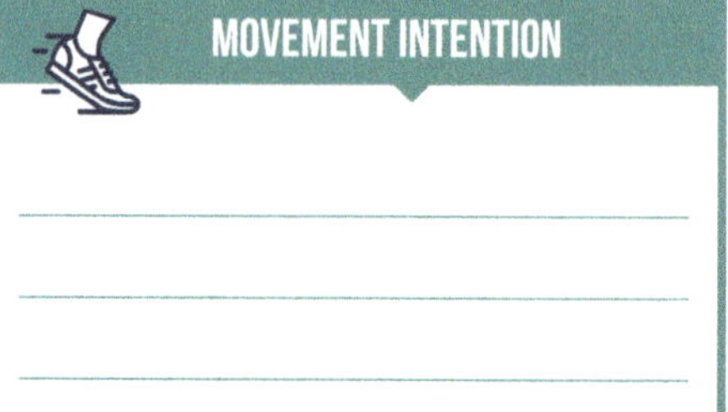

MEALS INTENTION

ON THE PLATE

OFF THE PLATE

MINDFUL AFFIRMATION:

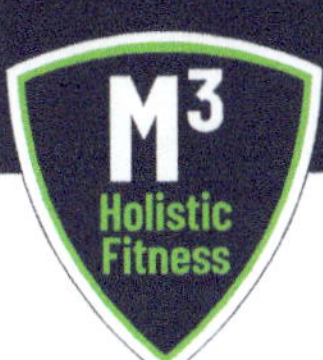

BEDTIME:

HYDRATION 1 2 3 4 5 6 7 8

WHAT DIDN'T WORK TODAY?:

MOVEMENT:

MEALS: ON OFF

TODAY'S WINS: 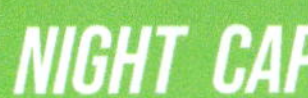

1

2

3

TODAY'S TAKE AWAY:

FOOD FOR THOUGHT FOR THE DAY:

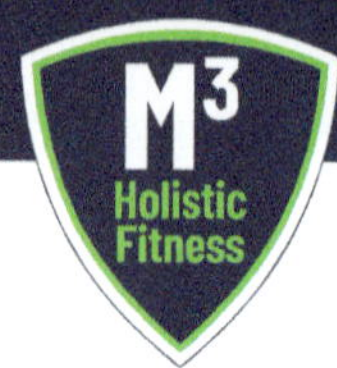

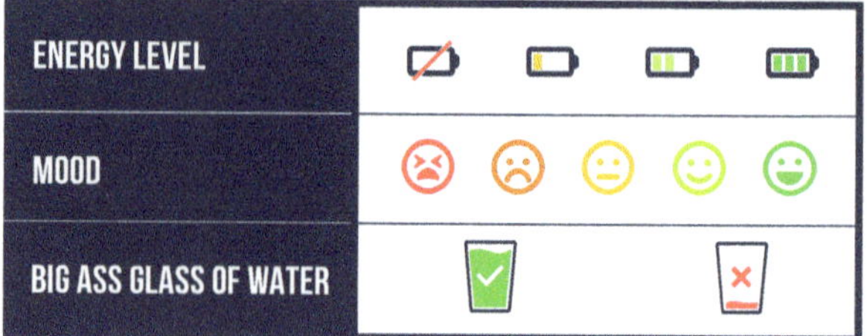

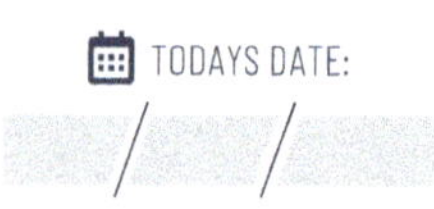

ENERGY LEVEL				
MOOD				
BIG ASS GLASS OF WATER				

I AM GRATEFUL FOR:

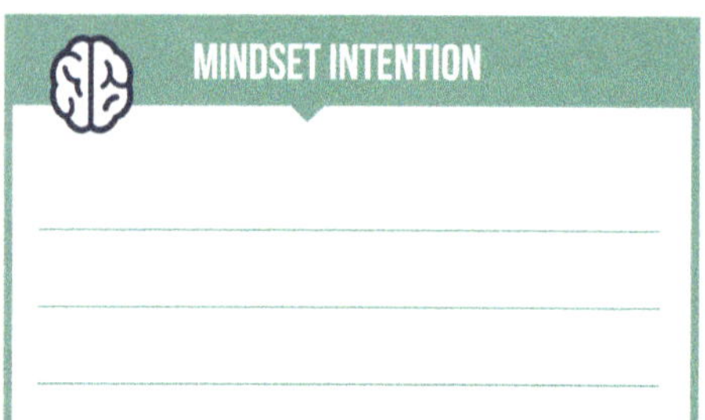

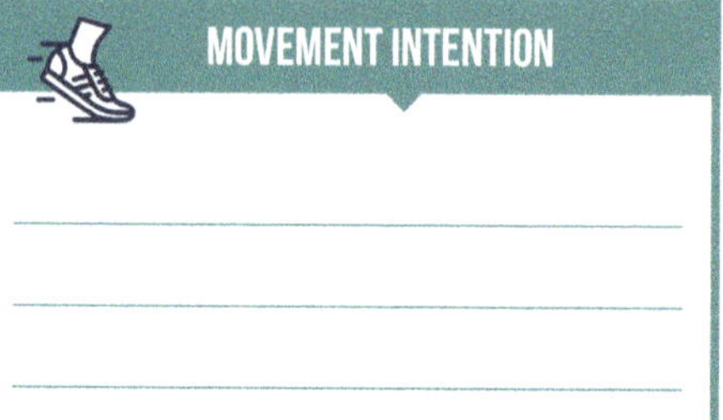

MINDFUL AFFIRMATION:

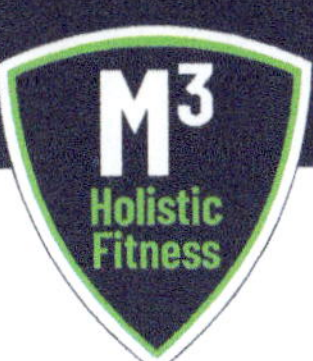

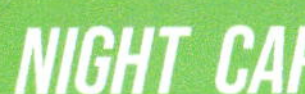

NIGHT CAP

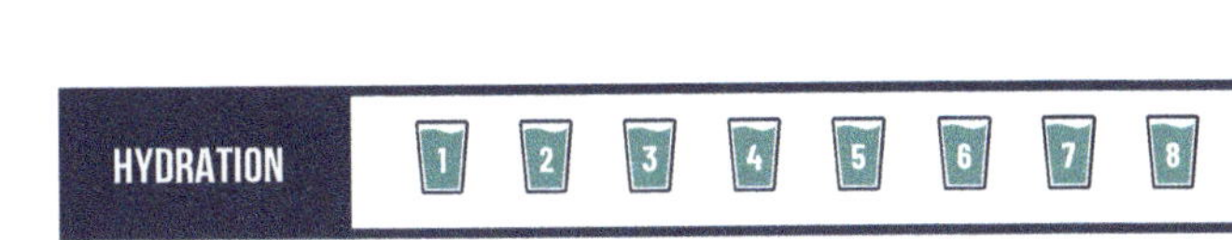

WHAT DIDN'T WORK TODAY?:

MOVEMENT: ☐

MEALS: ☐ ON ☐ OFF

TODAY'S WINS:

1

2

3

TODAY'S TAKE AWAY:

FOOD FOR THOUGHT FOR THE DAY:

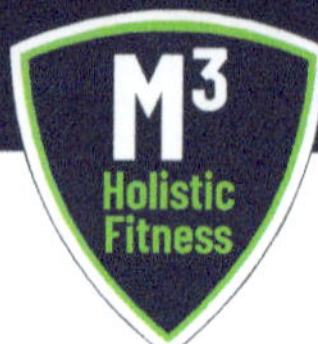

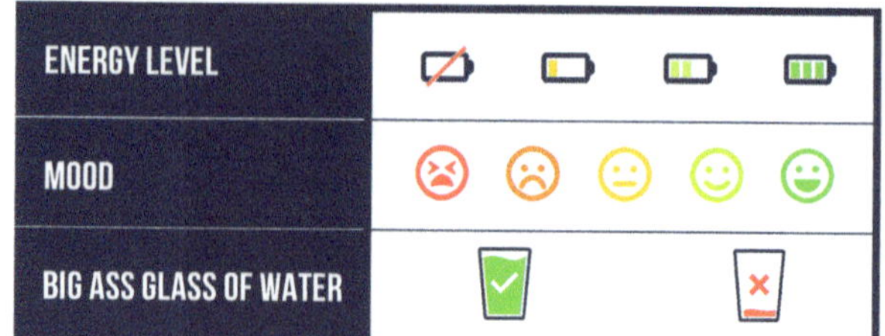

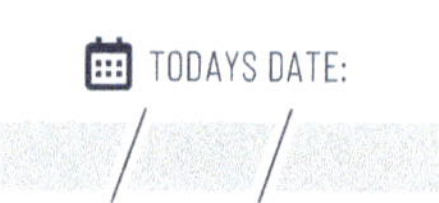

ENERGY LEVEL				
MOOD				
BIG ASS GLASS OF WATER				

I AM GRATEFUL FOR:

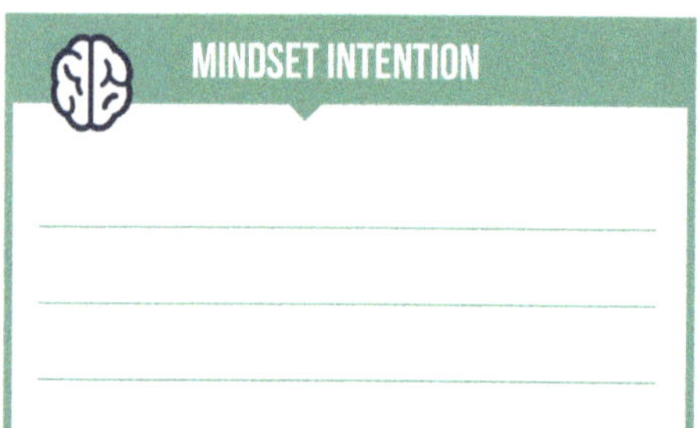

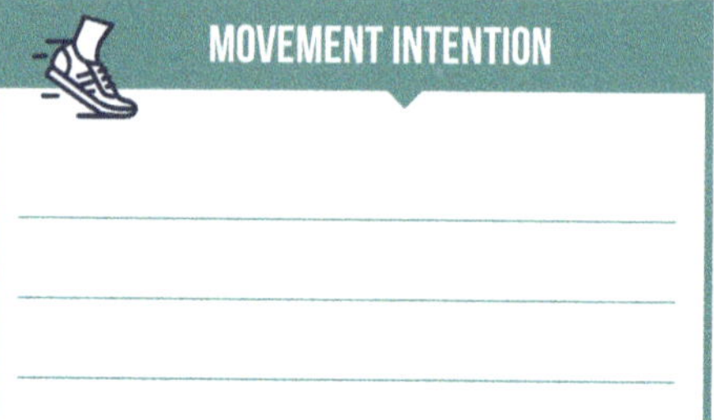

MEALS INTENTION

MINDFUL AFFIRMATION:

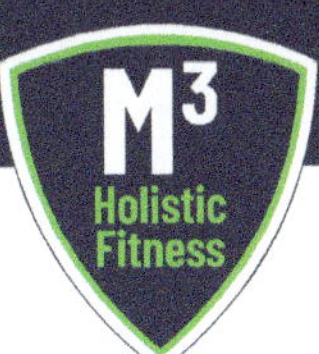

M³
Holistic Fitness

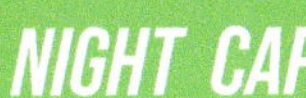
NIGHT CAP

BEDTIME:

HYDRATION 1 2 3 4 5 6 7 8

WHAT DIDN'T WORK TODAY?:

MOVEMENT: ☐

MEALS: ☐ ON ☐ OFF

TODAY'S WINS: 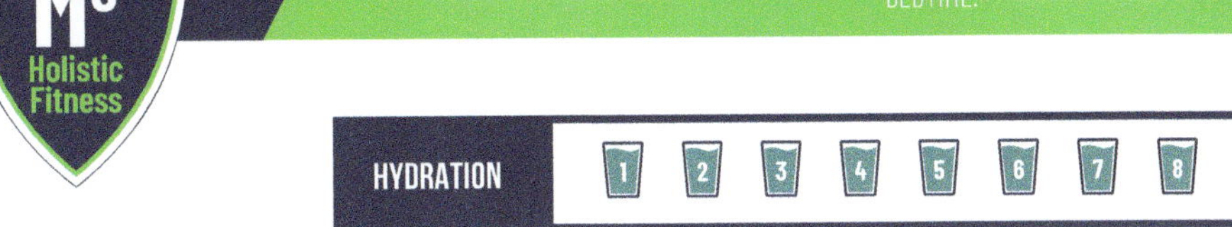

1

2

3

TODAY'S TAKE AWAY:

FOOD FOR THOUGHT FOR THE DAY:

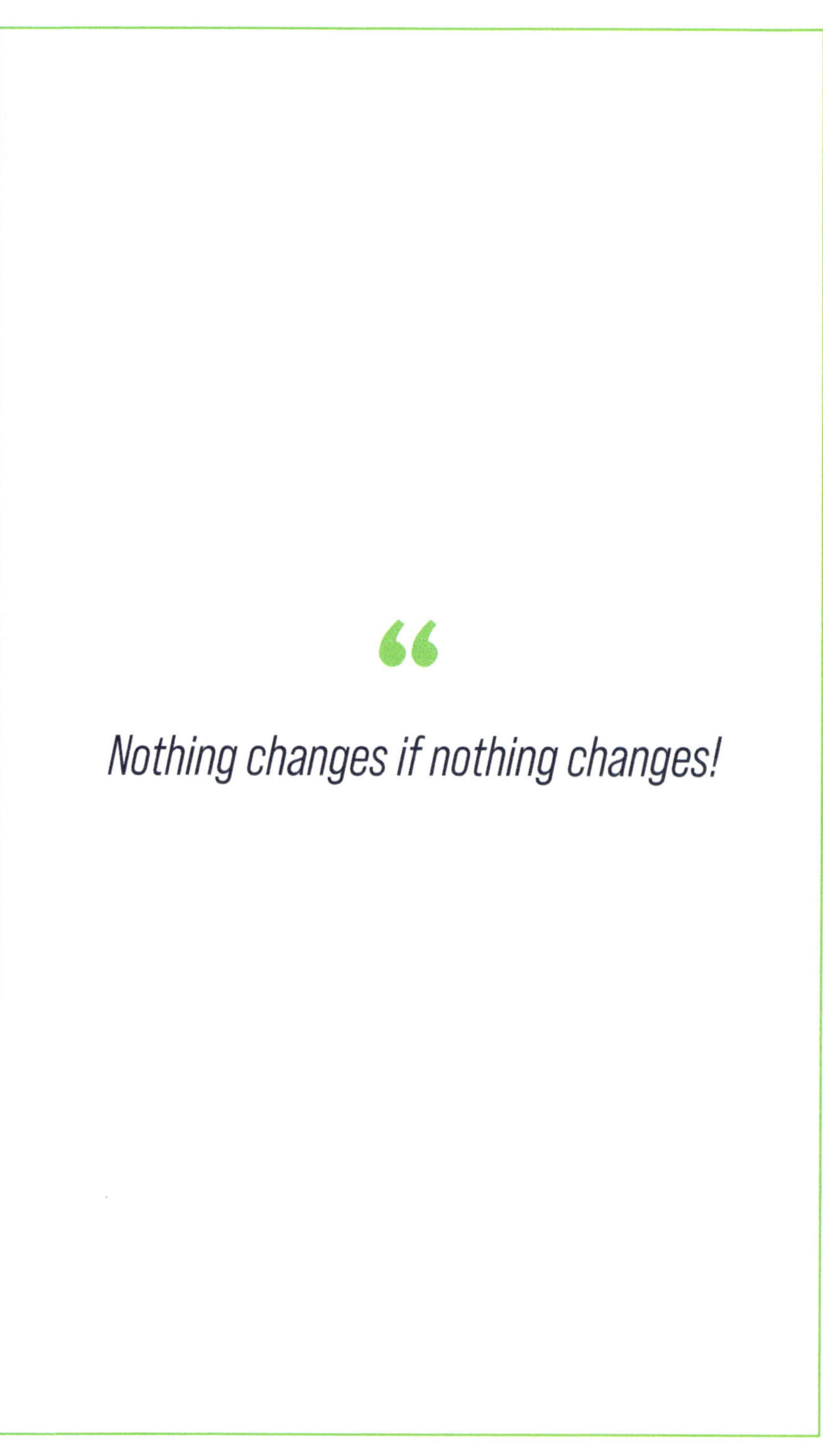

Nothing changes if nothing changes!

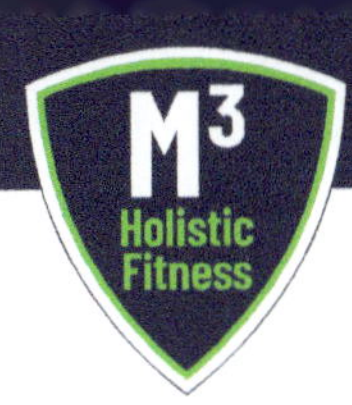

THIS WEEKS WINS:

THIS WEEKS TAKEAWAYS:

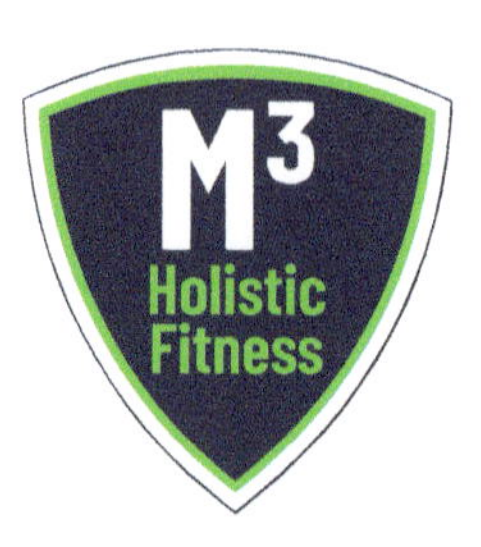

WEEK 2

90-DAY HOLISTIC FITNESS JOURNAL

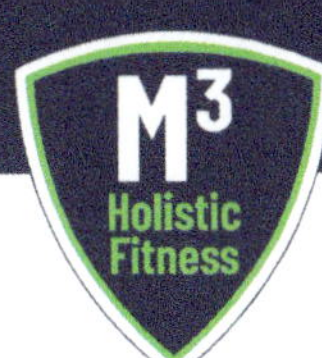

SATISFACTION

DISSATISFACTION

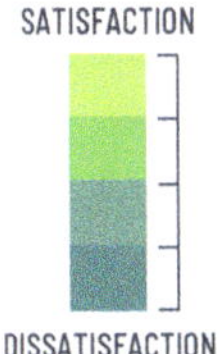

EXAMPLE

WHAT DOES YOUR LIFE LOOK LIKE?

1. Place a dot in each category to indicate your level of satisfaction within each area. A dot at the **center of the circle to indicate dissatisfaction**, or towards the **outer edge to indicate satisfaction**. Most people fall somewhere in between. (see example)

2. Connect the dots to see your **M₃ Circle of Life**.

3. Identify imbalances. Determine where to spend more time and energy to create balance. **This will help you create a better balance for your best Badass Life.**

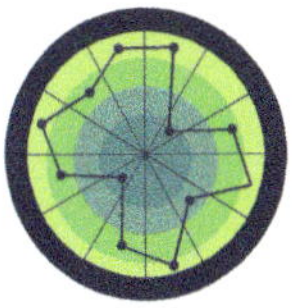

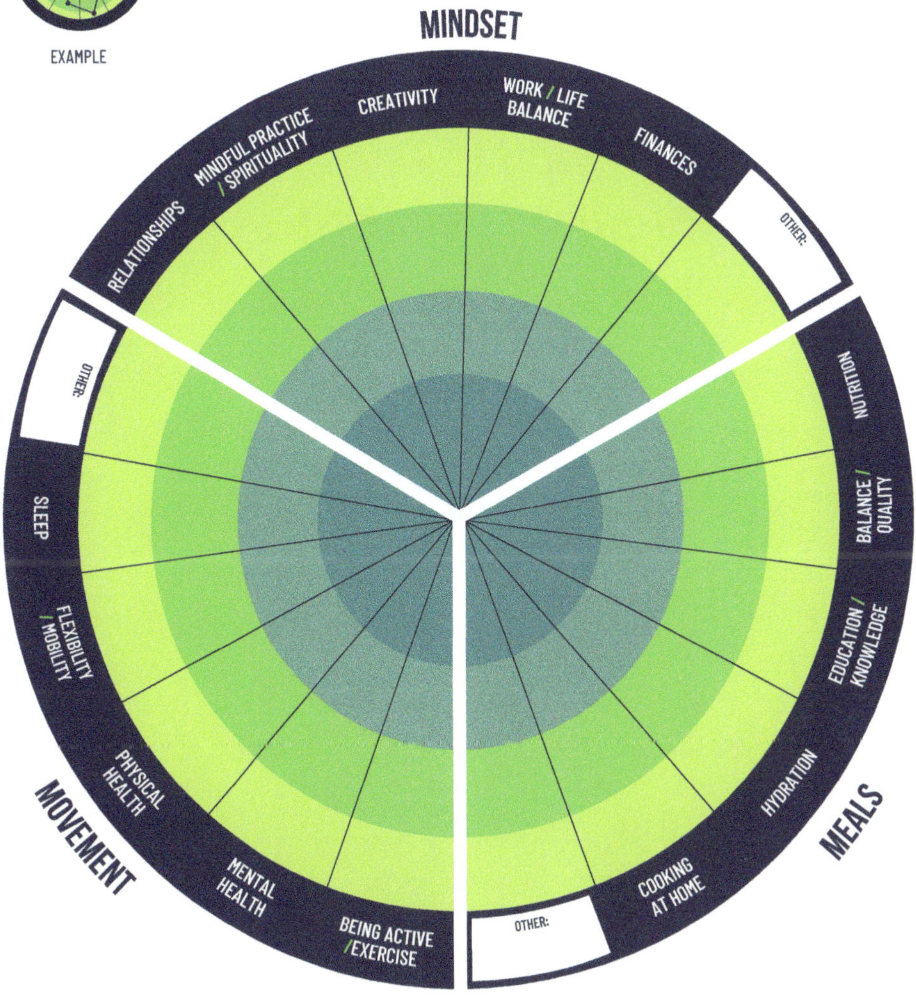

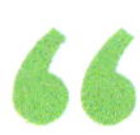

You're only as successful as your mindset.

M³
Holistic Fitness

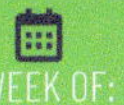

WEEK OF: ___ / ___ / ___

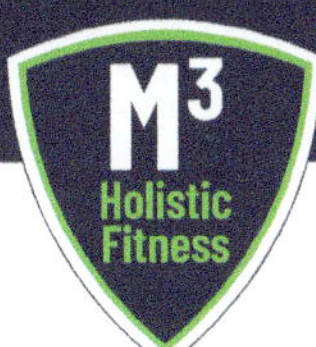

	MINDSET	MOVEMENT	MEALS ✓ ON THE PLATE	✓ OFF THE PLATE
MON				
TUES				
WEDS				
THURS				
FRI				
SAT				
SUN				

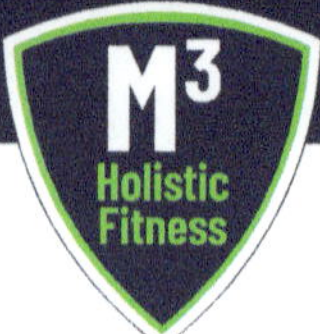
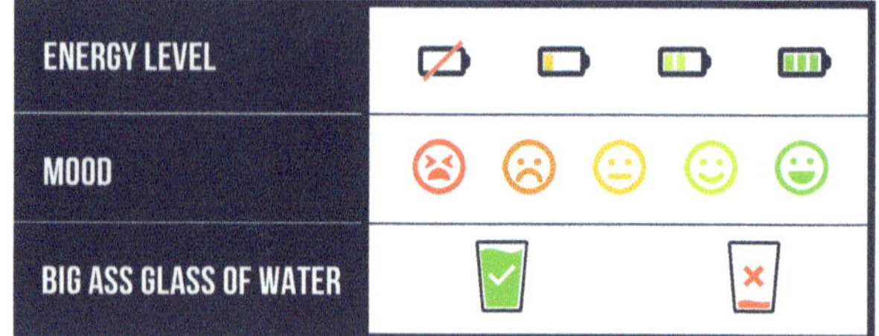

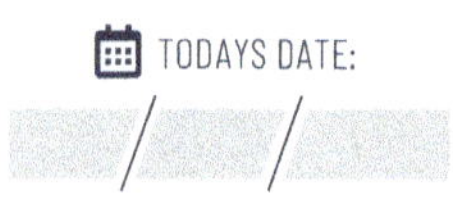

TODAYS DATE:

___ / ___ / ___

I AM GRATEFUL FOR:

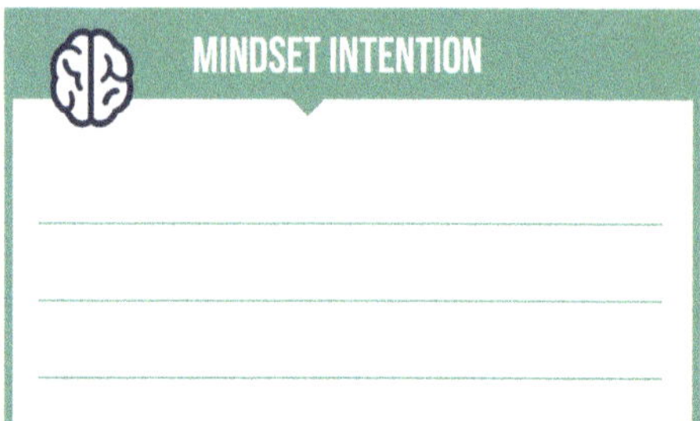

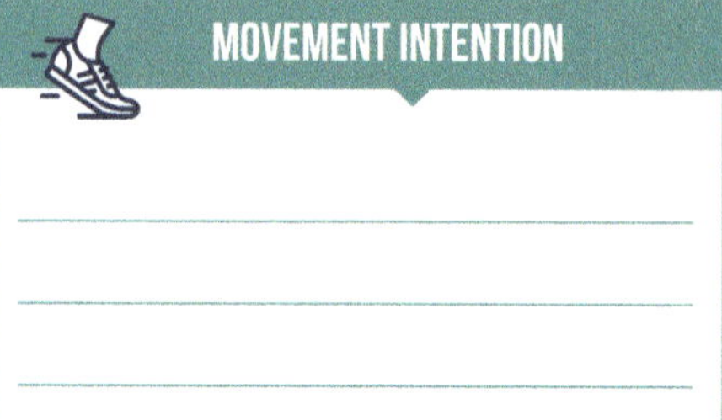

MINDFUL AFFIRMATION:

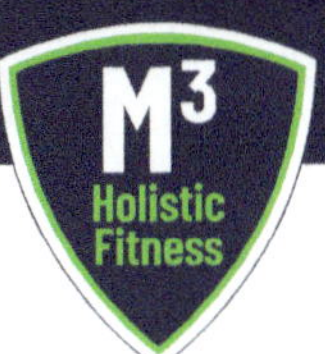

BEDTIME:

HYDRATION   1 2 3 4 5 6 7 8

WHAT DIDN'T WORK TODAY?:

MOVEMENT: ☐

MEALS: ☐ ON ☐ OFF

TODAY'S WINS:

1	2	3

TODAY'S TAKE AWAY:

FOOD FOR THOUGHT FOR THE DAY:

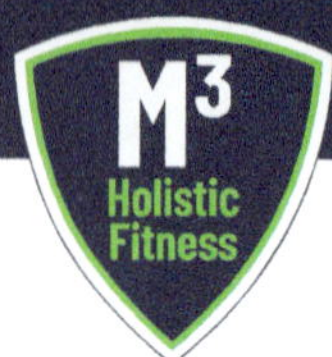

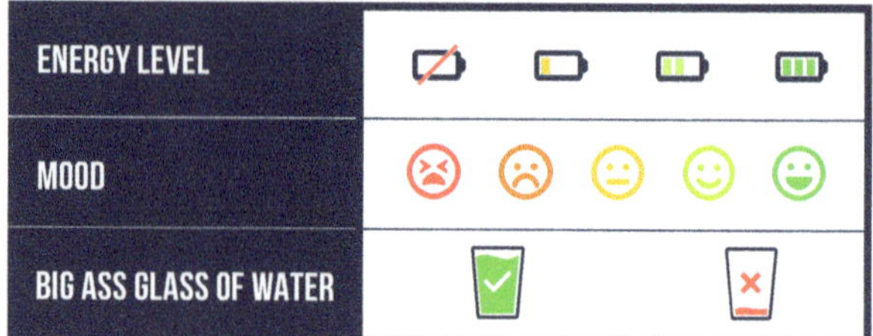

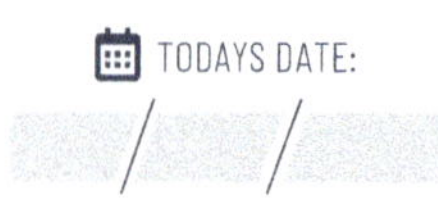

ENERGY LEVEL				
MOOD				
BIG ASS GLASS OF WATER				

I AM GRATEFUL FOR:

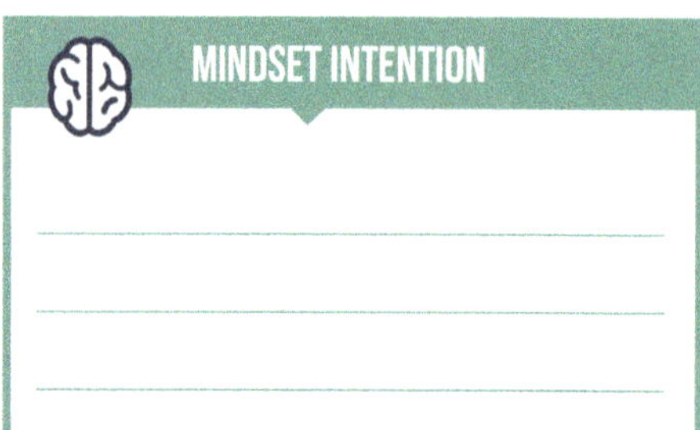

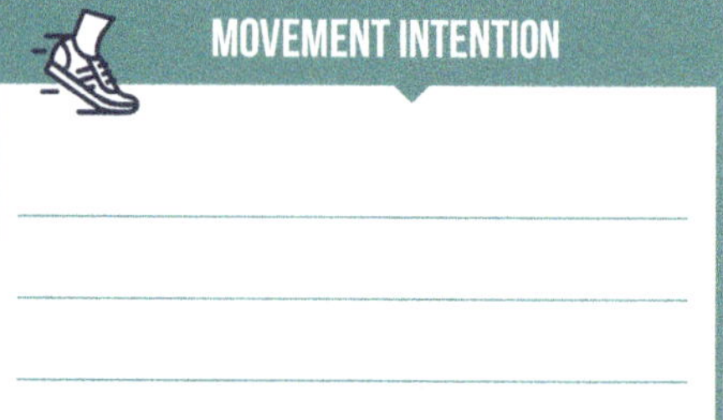

MINDFUL AFFIRMATION:

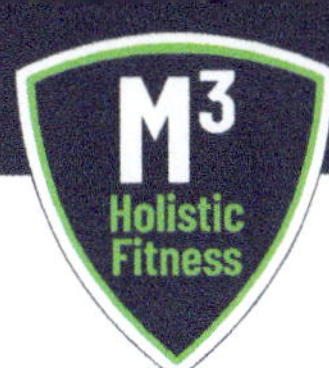

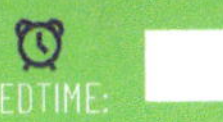

BEDTIME:

HYDRATION   1 2 3 4 5 6 7 8

WHAT DIDN'T WORK TODAY?:

____

____

MOVEMENT: ☐

MEALS: ☐ ON ☐ OFF

TODAY'S WINS: 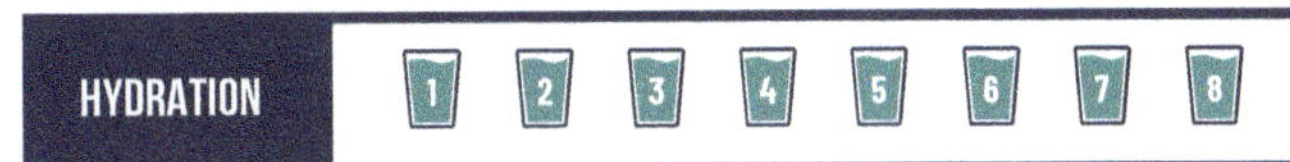

1

2

3

TODAY'S TAKE AWAY:

____

____

____

____

FOOD FOR THOUGHT FOR THE DAY:

____

____

____

____

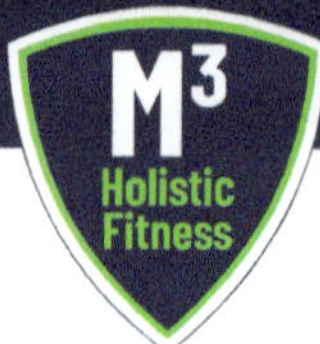

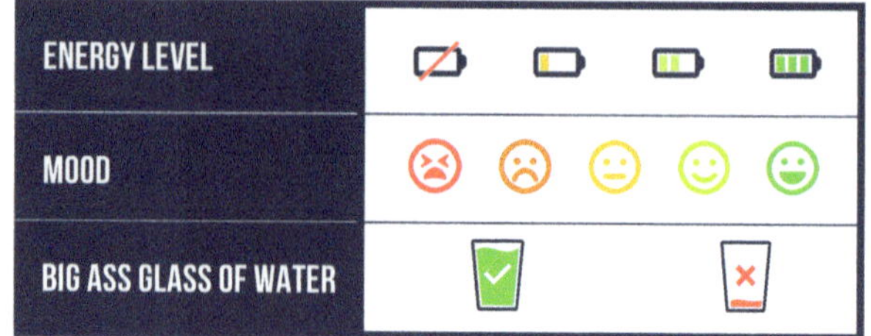

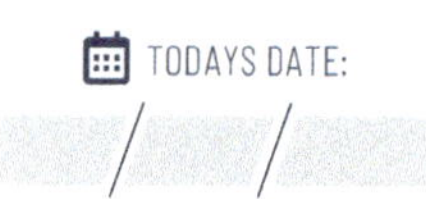

ENERGY LEVEL				
MOOD				
BIG ASS GLASS OF WATER				

___ / ___ / ___

I AM GRATEFUL FOR:

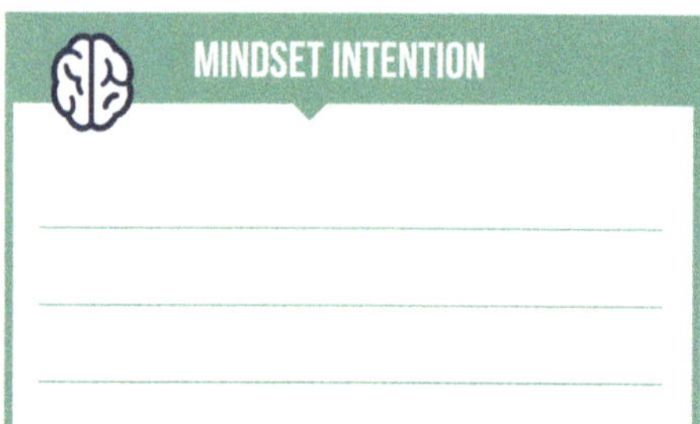

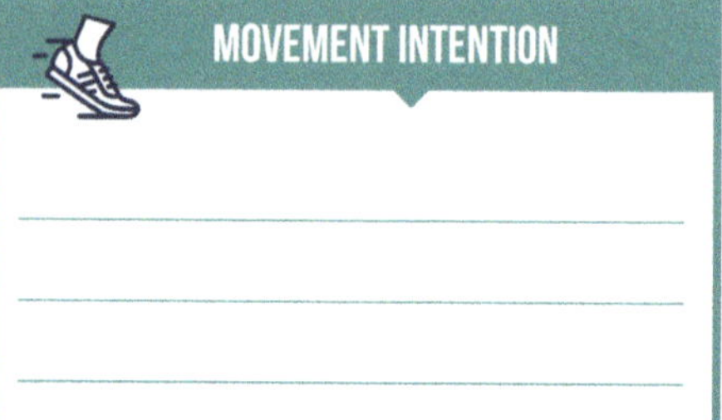

MEALS INTENTION

MINDFUL AFFIRMATION:

HYDRATION 1 2 3 4 5 6 7 8

WHAT DIDN'T WORK TODAY?:

MOVEMENT: ☐

MEALS: ☐ ON ☐ OFF

TODAY'S WINS: 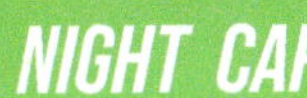

1

2

3

TODAY'S TAKE AWAY:

FOOD FOR THOUGHT FOR THE DAY:

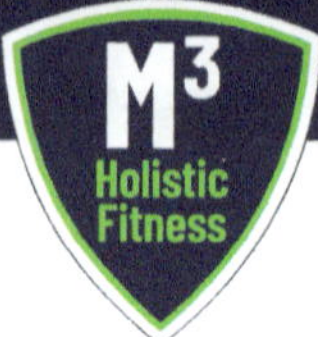

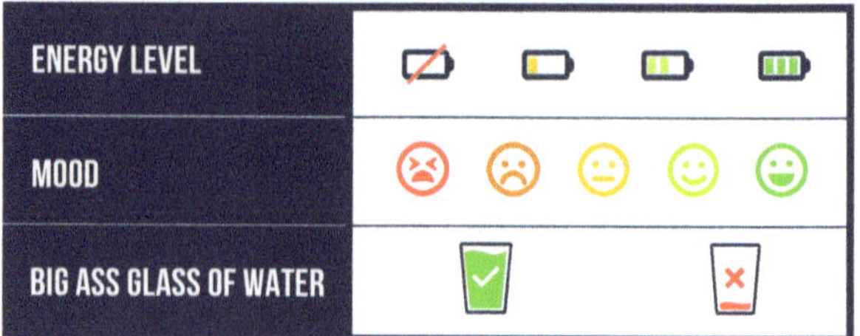

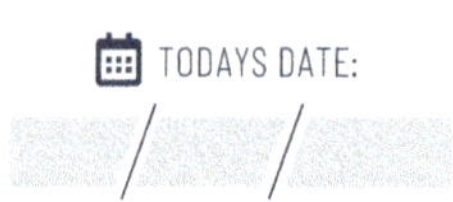
TODAYS DATE: ___ / ___ / ___

ENERGY LEVEL				
MOOD				
BIG ASS GLASS OF WATER				

I AM GRATEFUL FOR:

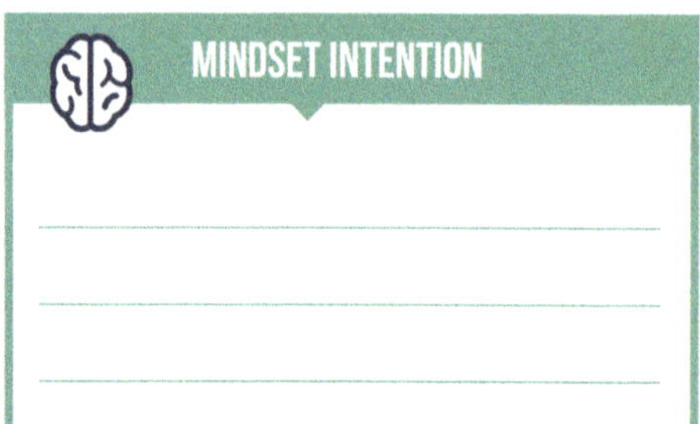

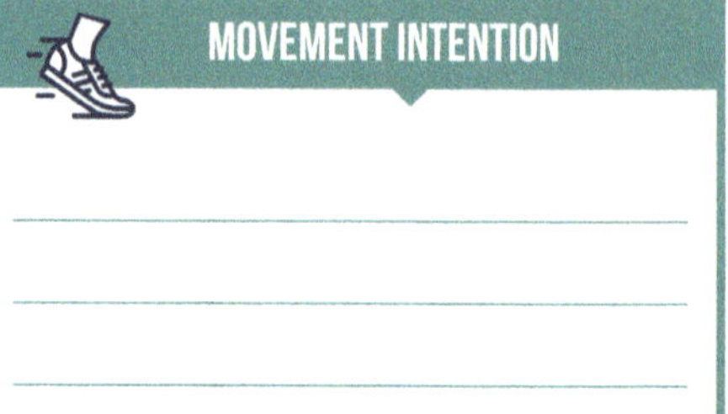

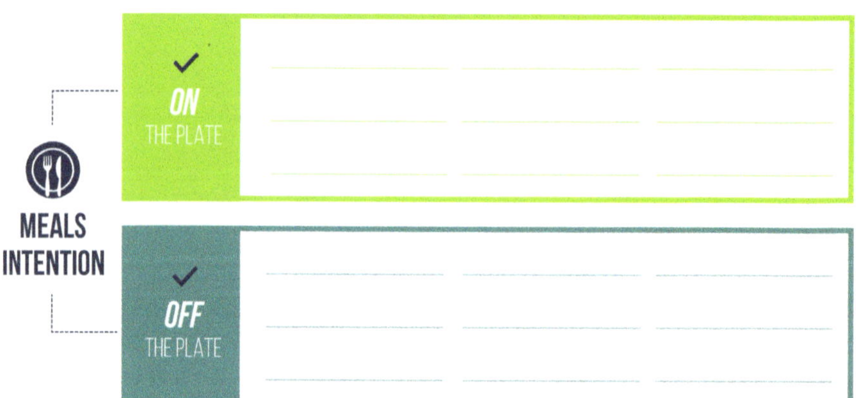

MINDFUL AFFIRMATION:

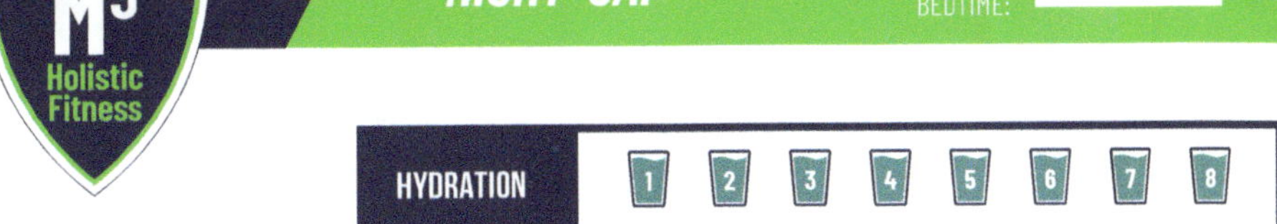

HYDRATION | 1 | 2 | 3 | 4 | 5 | 6 | 7 | 8 |

WHAT DIDN'T WORK TODAY?:

MOVEMENT: ☐

MEALS: ☐ ON ☐ OFF

TODAY'S WINS:

1

2

3

TODAY'S TAKE AWAY:

FOOD FOR THOUGHT FOR THE DAY:

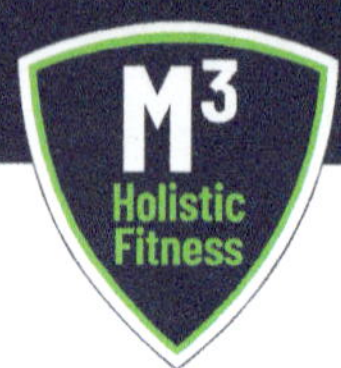

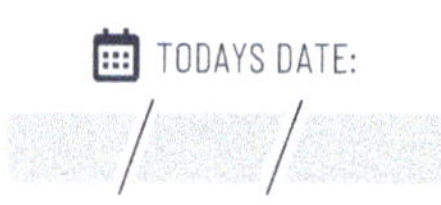

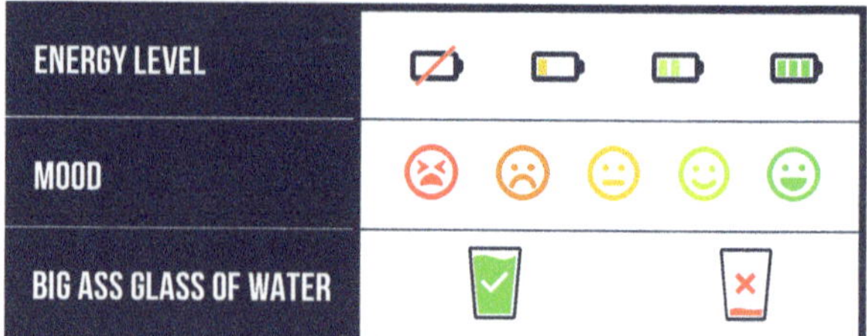

I AM GRATEFUL FOR:

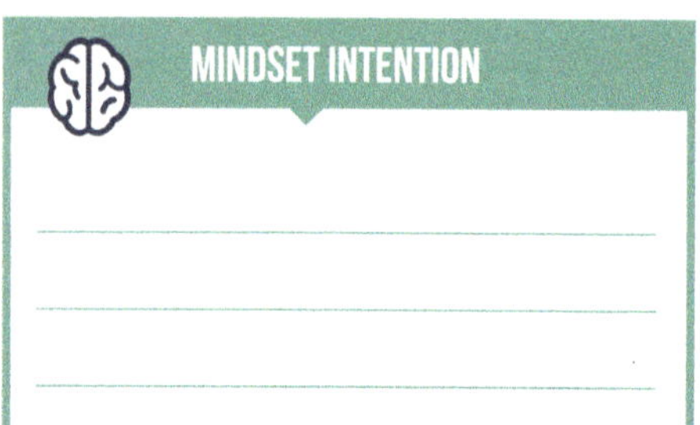

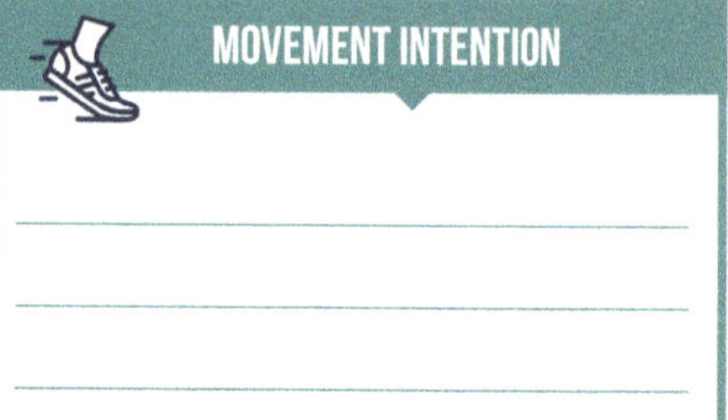

MINDFUL AFFIRMATION:

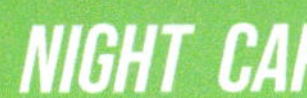
NIGHT CAP

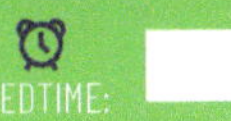
BEDTIME:

HYDRATION   1 2 3 4 5 6 7 8

WHAT DIDN'T WORK TODAY?:

MOVEMENT: ☐

MEALS: ☐ ON ☐ OFF

TODAY'S WINS: 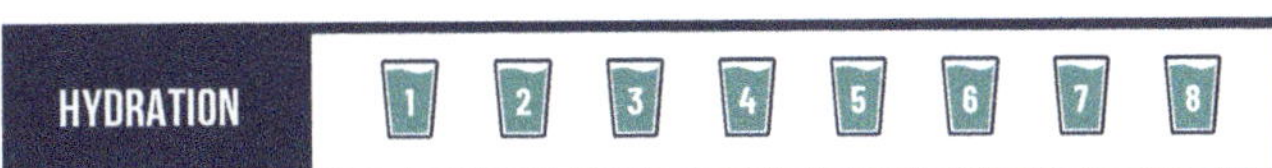

1
2
3

TODAY'S TAKE AWAY:

FOOD FOR THOUGHT FOR THE DAY:

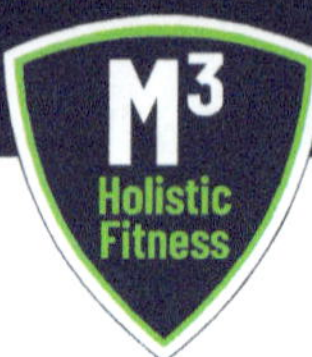

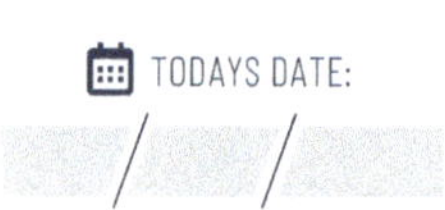

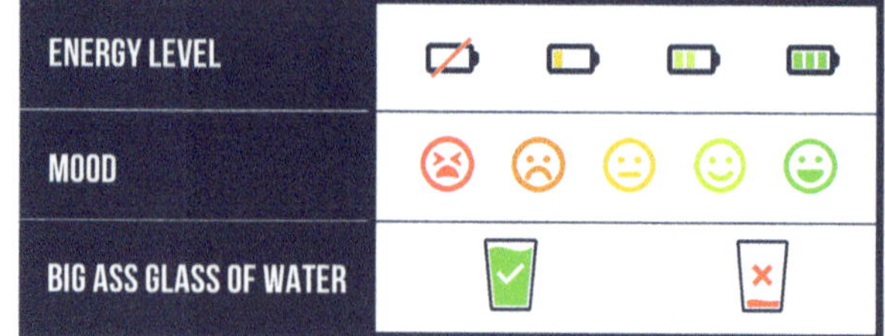

ENERGY LEVEL				
MOOD				
BIG ASS GLASS OF WATER				

I AM GRATEFUL FOR:

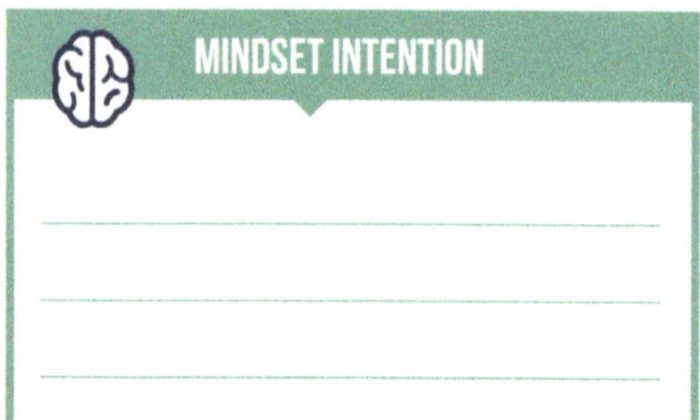

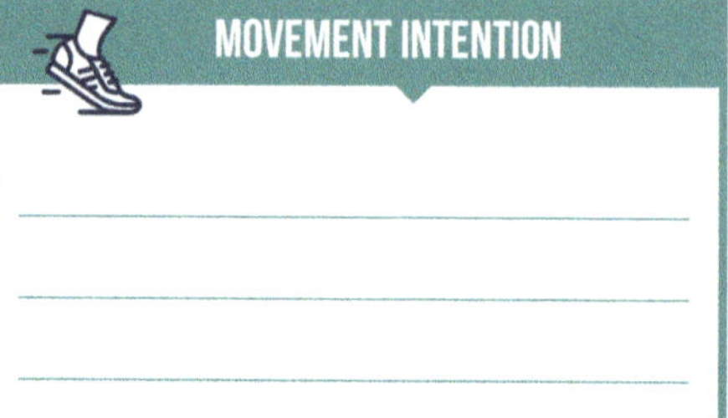

MINDFUL AFFIRMATION:

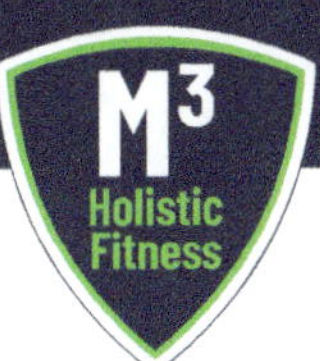

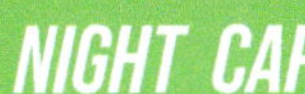

HYDRATION 1 2 3 4 5 6 7 8

WHAT DIDN'T WORK TODAY?:

MOVEMENT: MEALS: ON OFF

TODAY'S WINS:

1
2
3

TODAY'S TAKE AWAY:

FOOD FOR THOUGHT FOR THE DAY:

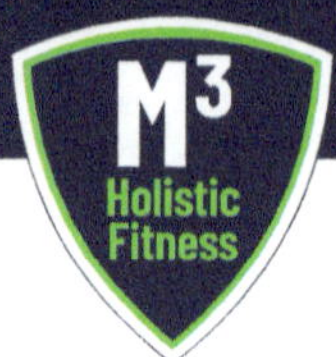

WAKE UP: SLEEP: Hrs

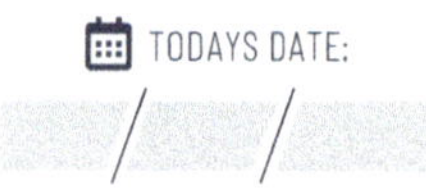

TODAYS DATE:

/   /

ENERGY LEVEL				
MOOD				
BIG ASS GLASS OF WATER				

I AM GRATEFUL FOR:

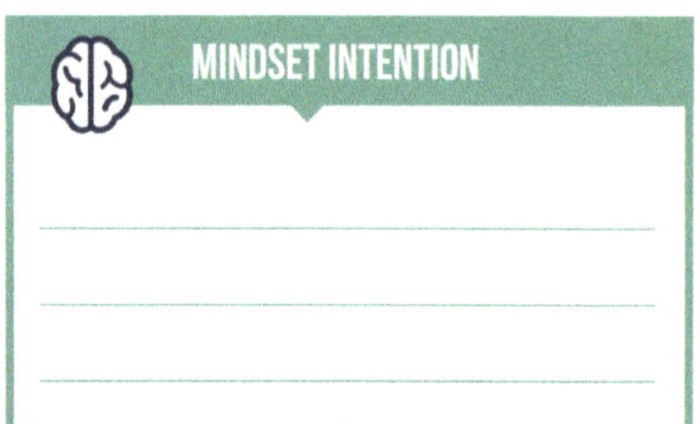

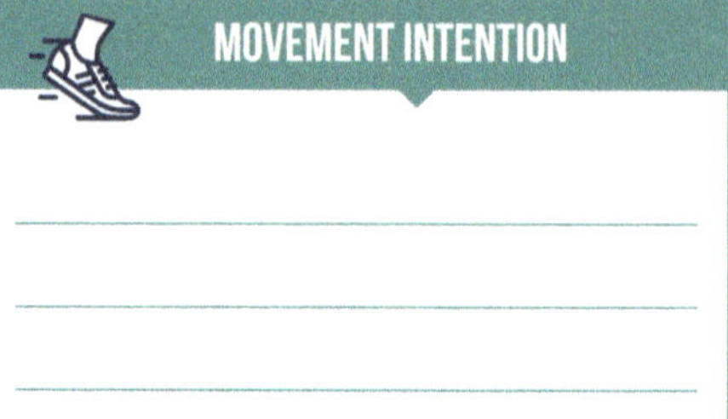

MINDFUL AFFIRMATION:

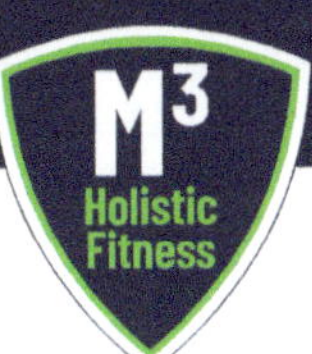

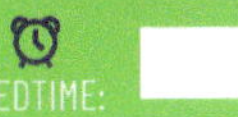

BEDTIME:

HYDRATION 1 2 3 4 5 6 7 8

WHAT DIDN'T WORK TODAY?:

MOVEMENT:

MEALS: ON OFF

TODAY'S WINS: 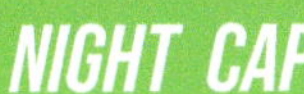

1

2

3

TODAY'S TAKE AWAY:

FOOD FOR THOUGHT FOR THE DAY:

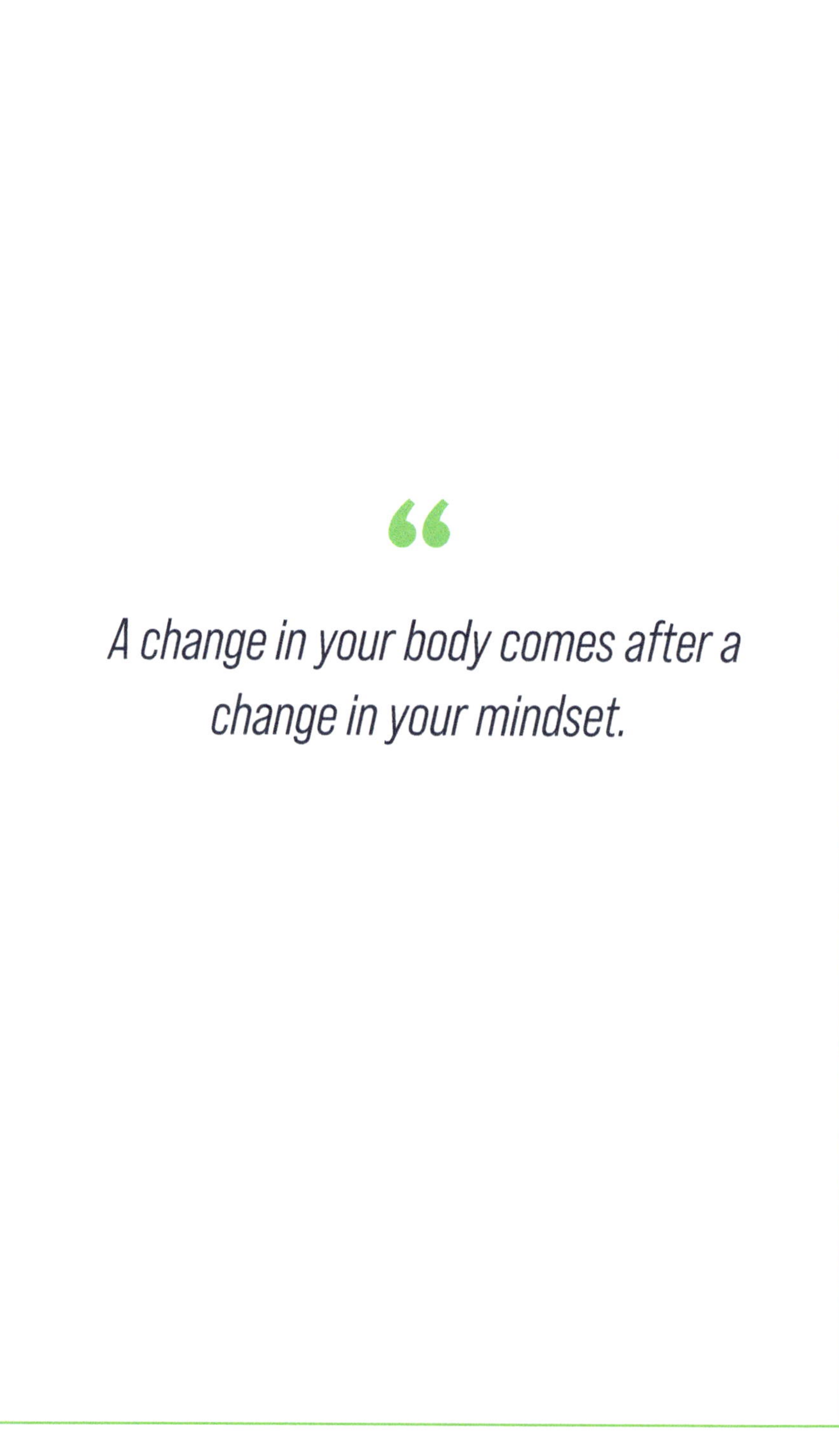

A change in your body comes after a change in your mindset.

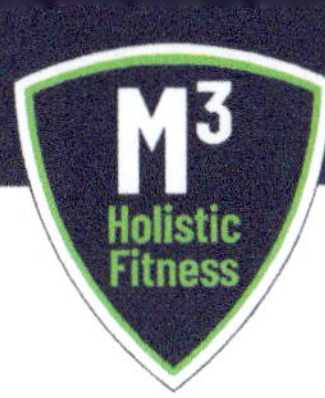

THIS WEEKS WINS:

THIS WEEKS TAKEAWAYS:

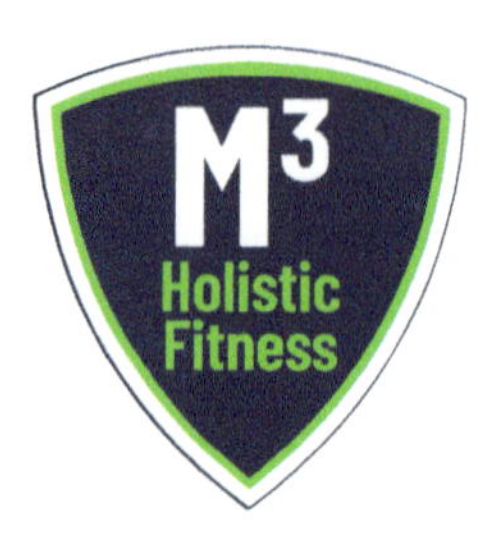

WEEK 3

90-DAY HOLISTIC FITNESS JOURNAL

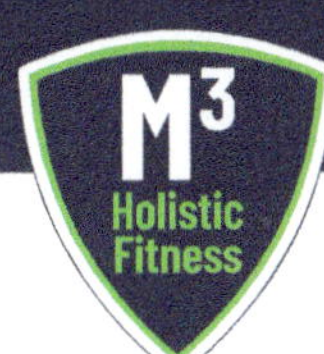

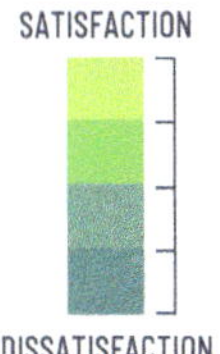

SATISFACTION

DISSATISFACTION

EXAMPLE

WHAT DOES YOUR LIFE LOOK LIKE?

1. Place a dot in each category to indicate your level of satisfaction within each area. A dot at the **center of the circle to indicate dissatisfaction,** or towards the **outer edge to indicate satisfaction.** Most people fall somewhere in between. (see example)

2. Connect the dots to see your **M3 Circle of Life.**

3. Identify imbalances. Determine where to spend more time and energy to create balance. **This will help you create a better balance for your best Badass Life.**

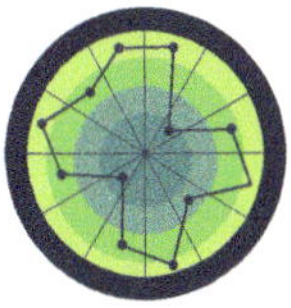

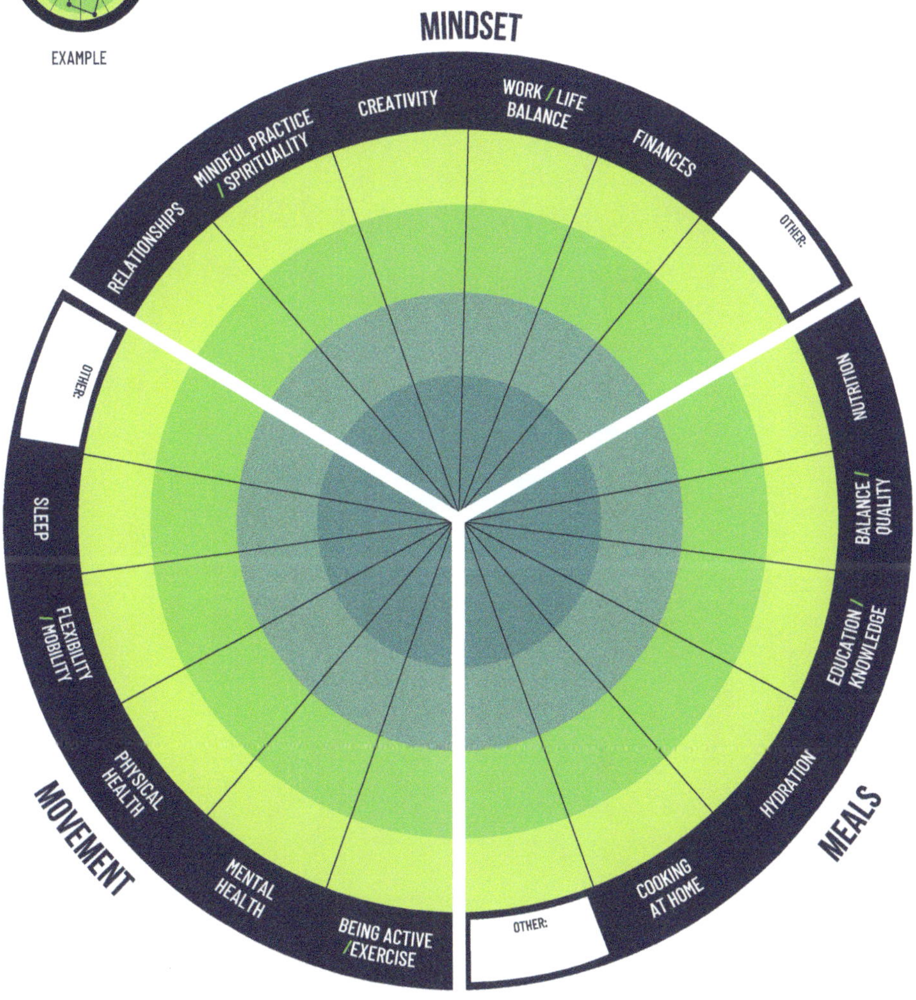

*Your body hears everything
your mind says.*

-Naomi Judd

	MINDSET	MOVEMENT	MEALS ✓ ON THE PLATE	✓ OFF THE PLATE
MON				
TUES				
WEDS				
THURS				
FRI				
SAT				
SUN				

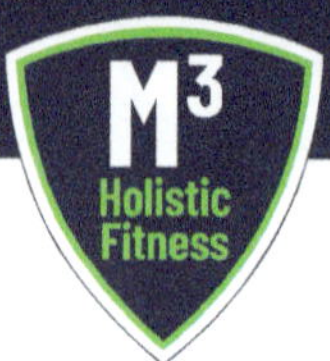

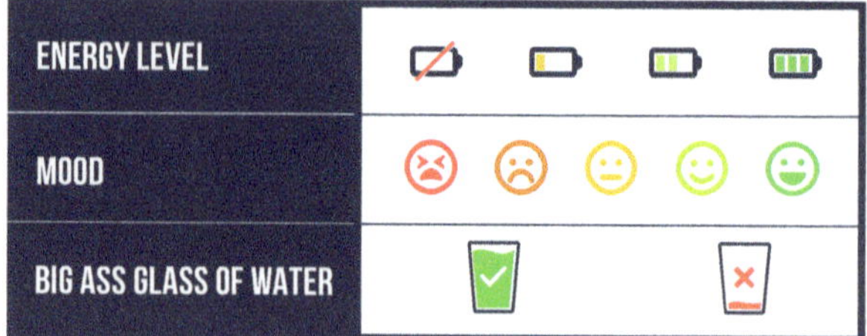

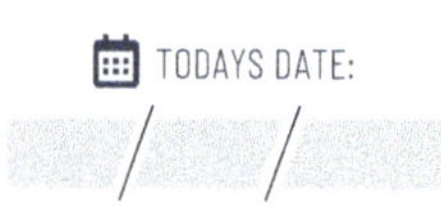

I AM GRATEFUL FOR:

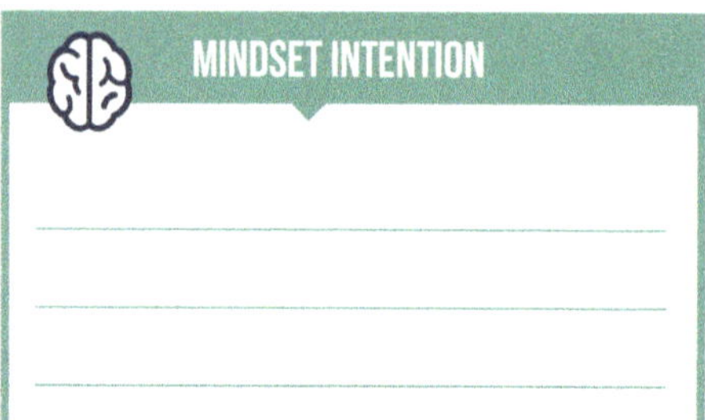

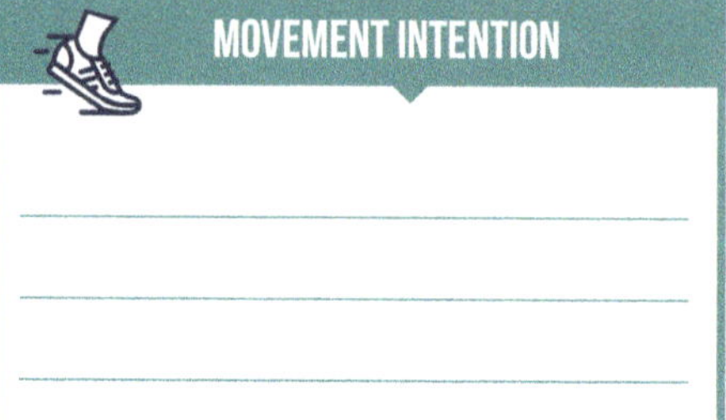

MINDFUL AFFIRMATION:

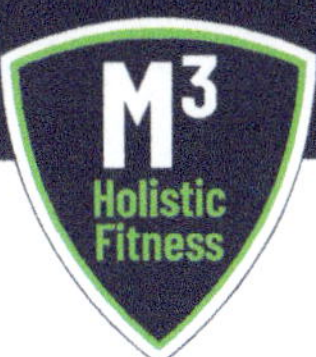

NIGHT CAP

HYDRATION 1 2 3 4 5 6 7 8

WHAT DIDN'T WORK TODAY?:

MOVEMENT: ☐

MEALS: ☐ ON ☐ OFF

TODAY'S WINS: 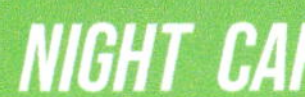

1
2
3

TODAY'S TAKE AWAY:

FOOD FOR THOUGHT FOR THE DAY:

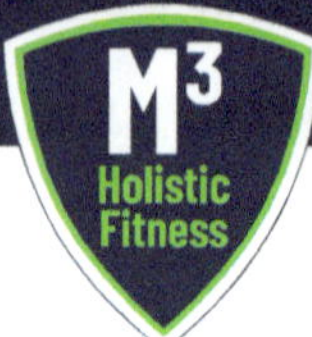

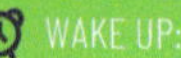

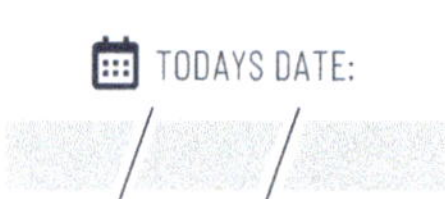

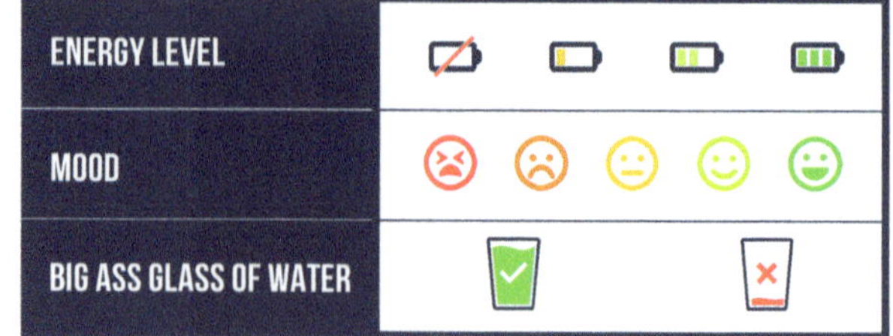

TODAYS DATE:

I AM GRATEFUL FOR:

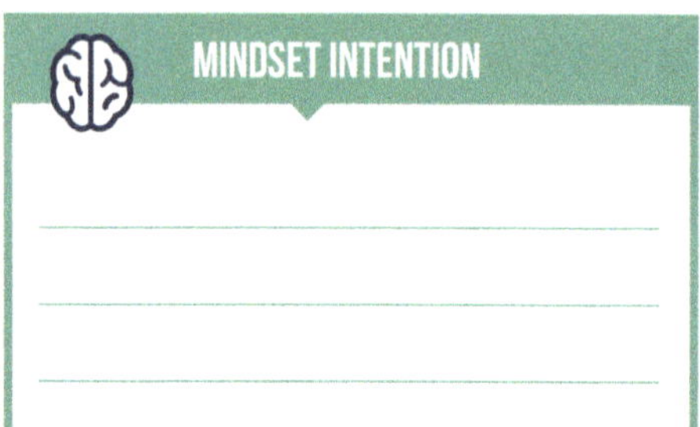

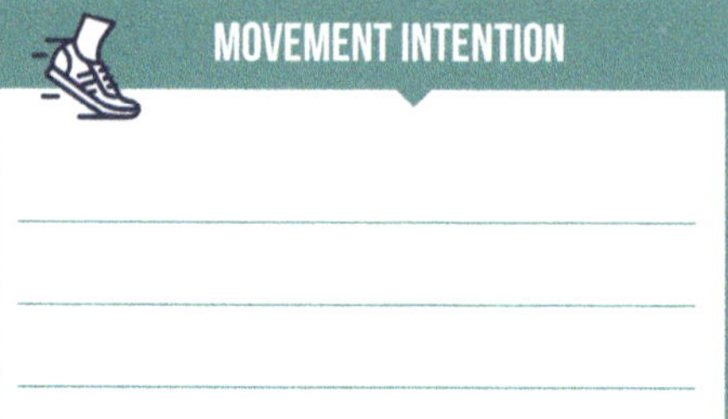

MINDFUL AFFIRMATION:

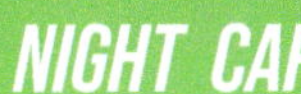

NIGHT CAP

BEDTIME:

HYDRATION 1 2 3 4 5 6 7 8

WHAT DIDN'T WORK TODAY?:

MOVEMENT: ☐

MEALS: ☐ ON ☐ OFF

TODAY'S WINS:

1

2

3

TODAY'S TAKE AWAY:

FOOD FOR THOUGHT FOR THE DAY:

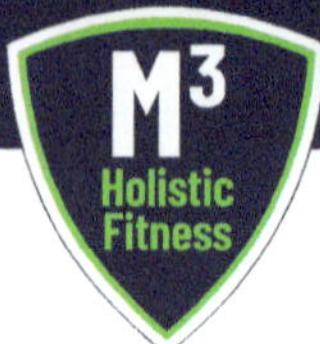

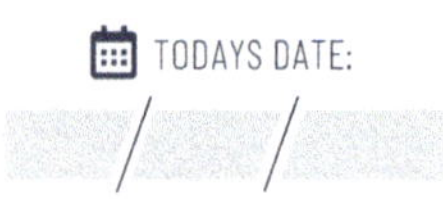

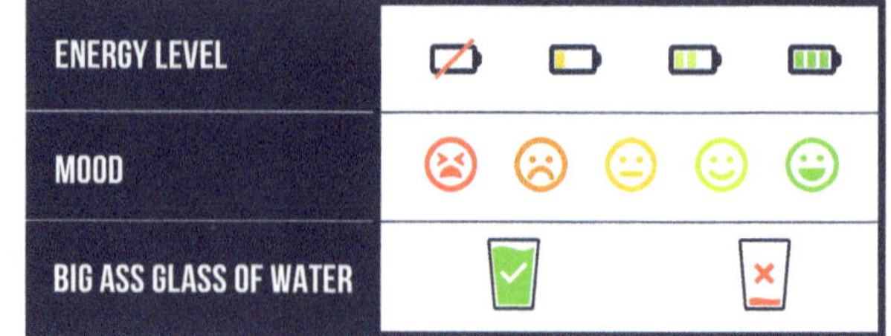

I AM GRATEFUL FOR:

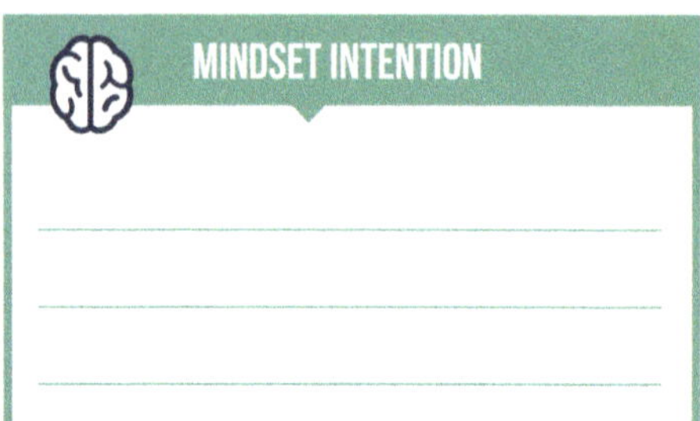

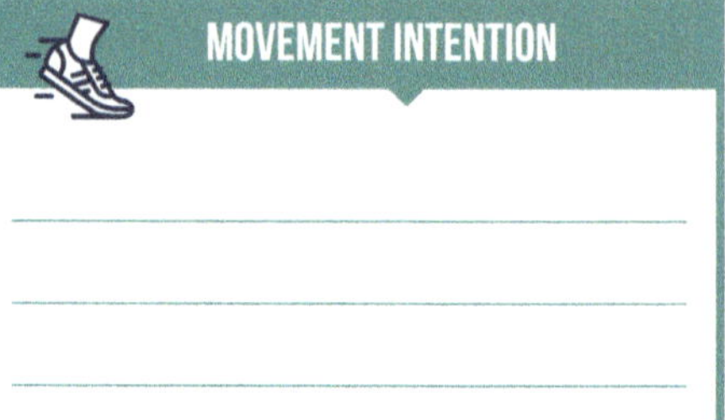

MINDFUL AFFIRMATION:

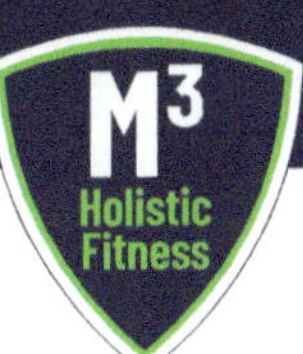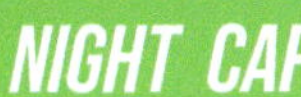

NIGHT CAP

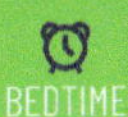
BEDTIME:

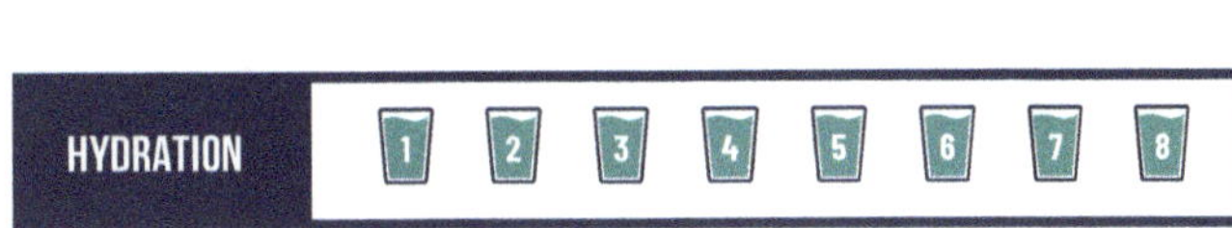

WHAT DIDN'T WORK TODAY?:

MOVEMENT: ☐

MEALS: ☐ ON ☐ OFF

TODAY'S WINS:

1

2

3

TODAY'S TAKE AWAY:

FOOD FOR THOUGHT FOR THE DAY:

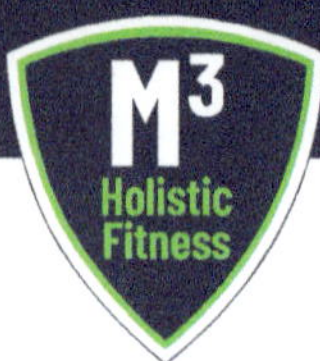

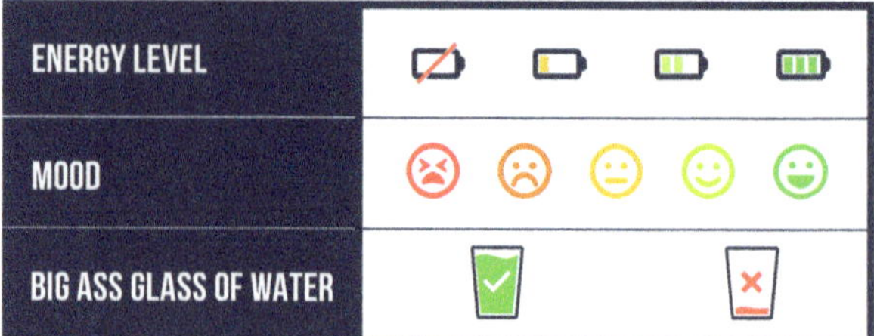

ENERGY LEVEL				
MOOD				
BIG ASS GLASS OF WATER				

I AM GRATEFUL FOR:

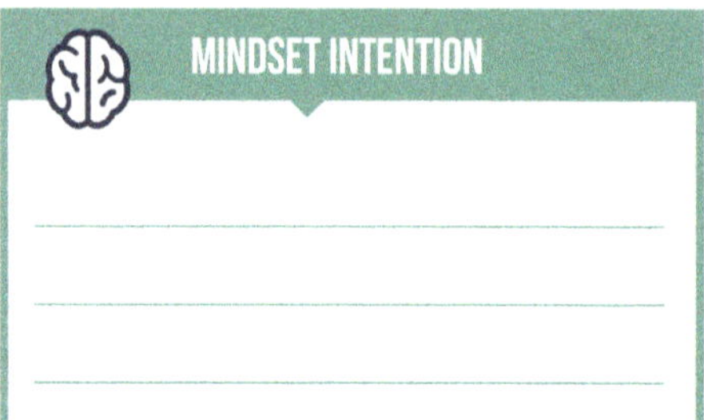

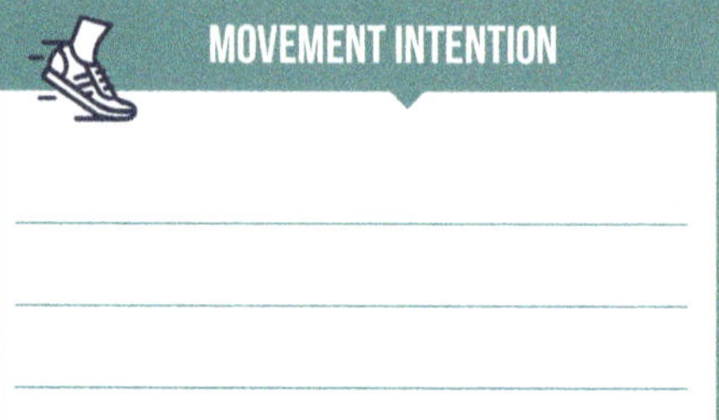

MINDFUL AFFIRMATION:

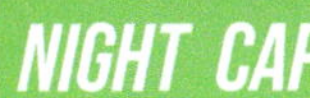

BEDTIME:

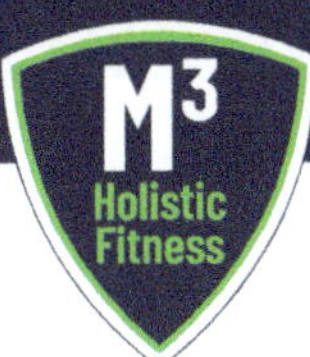

M³ Holistic Fitness

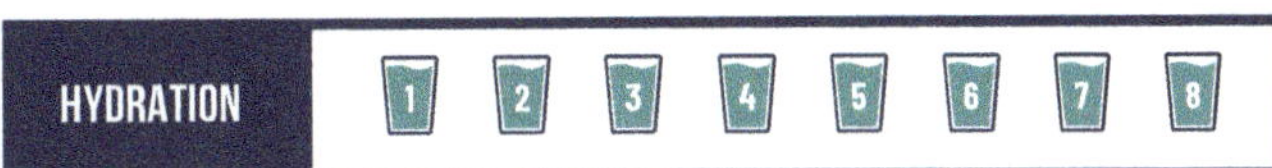

HYDRATION 1 2 3 4 5 6 7 8

WHAT DIDN'T WORK TODAY?:

MOVEMENT: ☐

MEALS: ☐ ON ☐ OFF

TODAY'S WINS:

1

2

3

TODAY'S TAKE AWAY:

FOOD FOR THOUGHT FOR THE DAY:

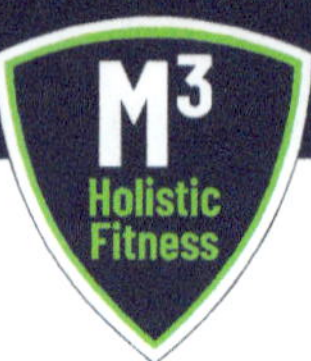

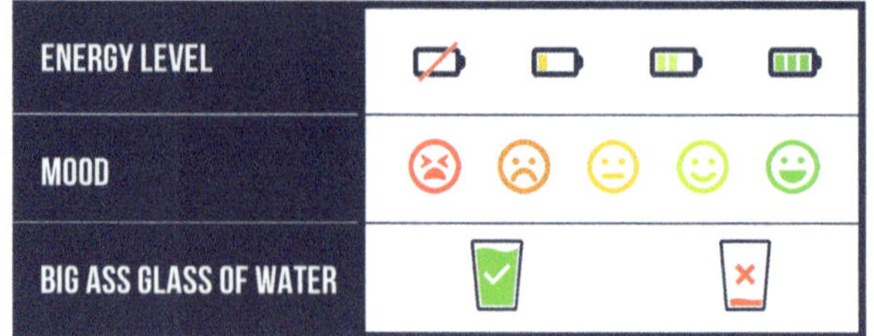

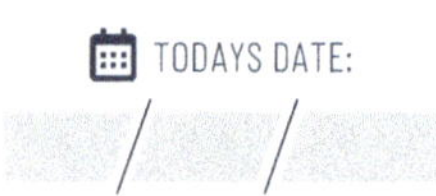

ENERGY LEVEL				
MOOD				
BIG ASS GLASS OF WATER				

I AM GRATEFUL FOR:

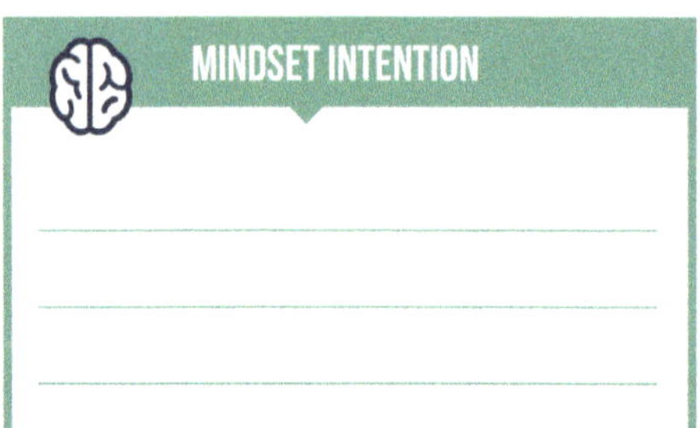

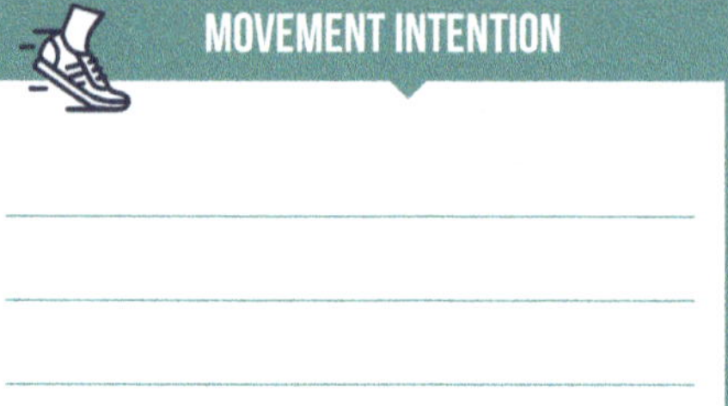

MEALS INTENTION

MINDFUL AFFIRMATION:

NIGHT CAP

BEDTIME:

HYDRATION 1 2 3 4 5 6 7 8

WHAT DIDN'T WORK TODAY?:

MOVEMENT: ☐

MEALS: ☐ ON ☐ OFF

TODAY'S WINS:

1

2

3

TODAY'S TAKE AWAY:

FOOD FOR THOUGHT FOR THE DAY:

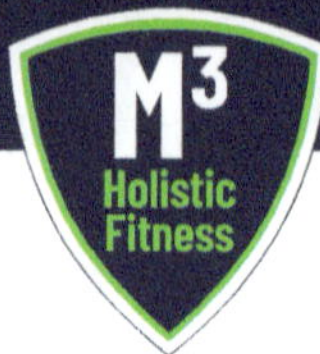

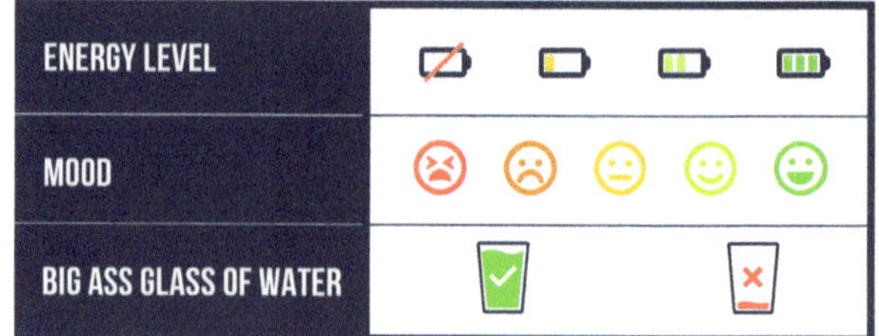

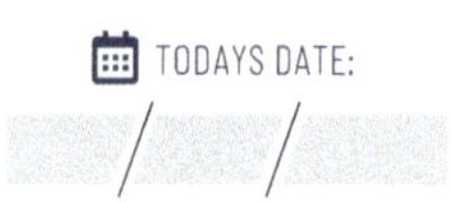

I AM GRATEFUL FOR:

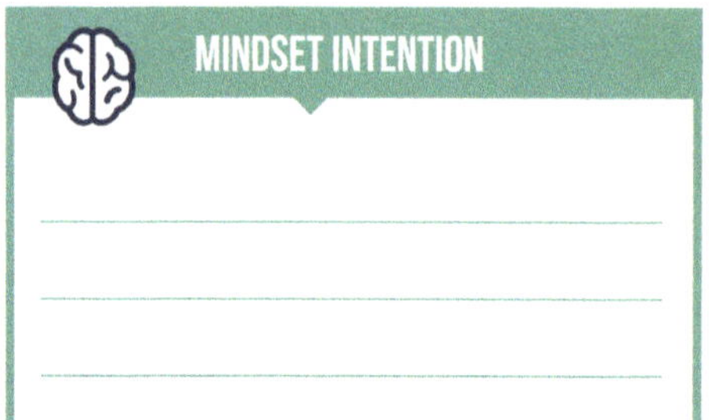

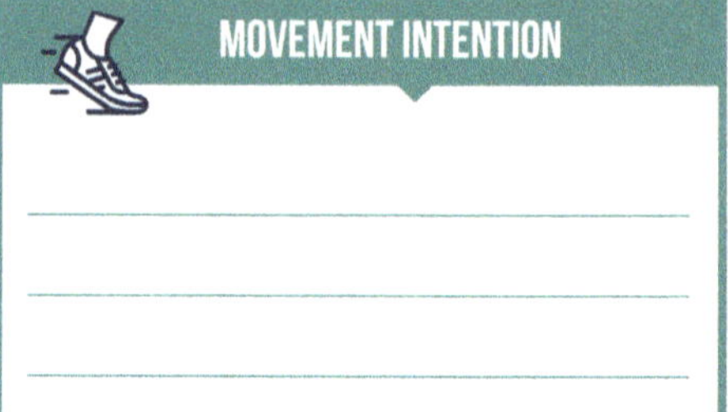

MINDFUL AFFIRMATION:

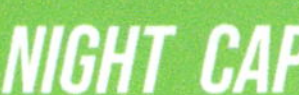

BEDTIME:

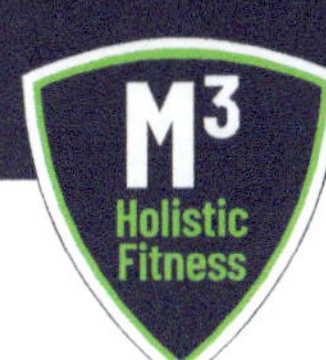

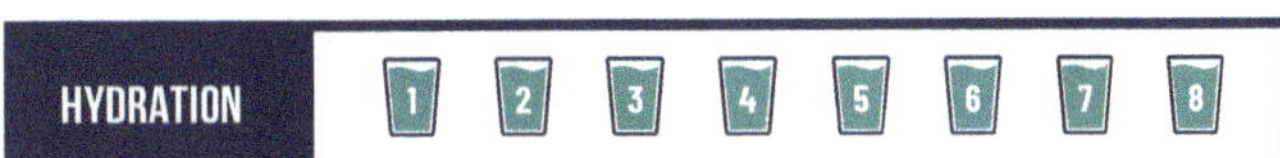

HYDRATION 1 2 3 4 5 6 7 8

WHAT DIDN'T WORK TODAY?:

MOVEMENT: ☐

MEALS: ☐ ON ☐ OFF

TODAY'S WINS:

1

2

3

TODAY'S TAKE AWAY:

FOOD FOR THOUGHT FOR THE DAY:

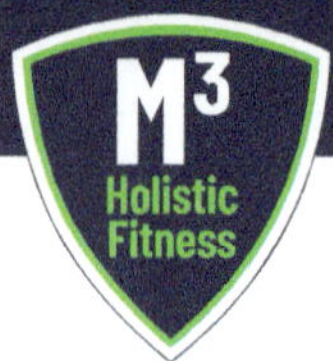

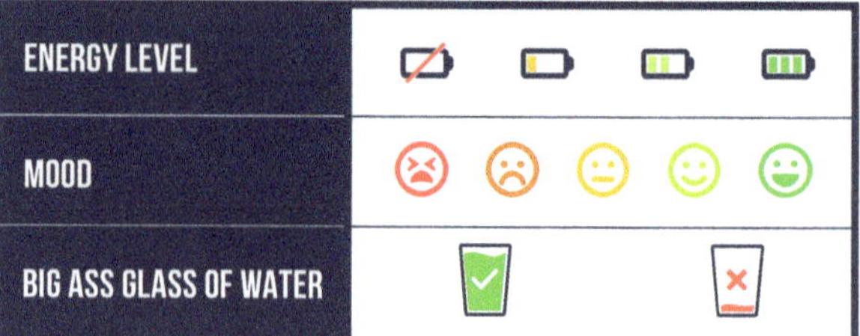

ENERGY LEVEL				
MOOD				
BIG ASS GLASS OF WATER		✓		✗

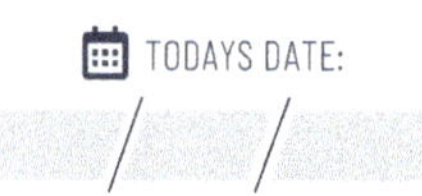
TODAYS DATE:
___ / ___ / ___

I AM GRATEFUL FOR:

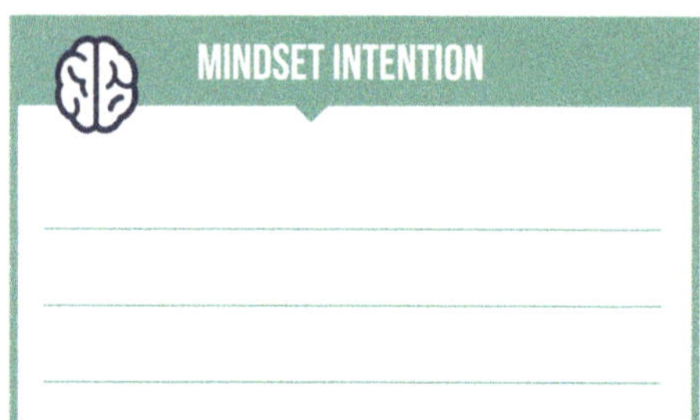

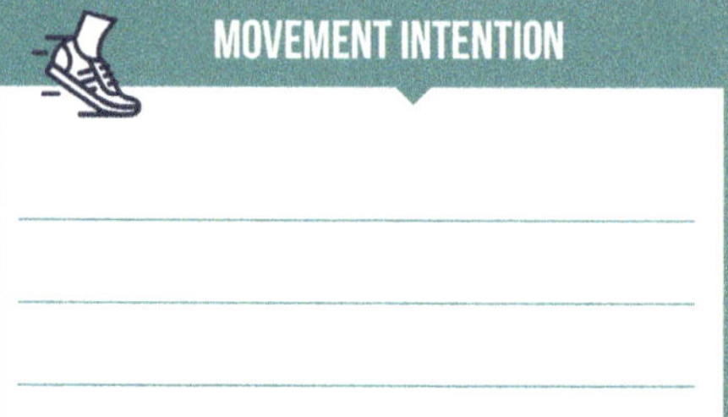

MEALS INTENTION

MINDFUL AFFIRMATION:

HYDRATION   1 2 3 4 5 6 7 8

WHAT DIDN'T WORK TODAY?:

MOVEMENT: ☐

MEALS: ☐ ON   ☐ OFF

TODAY'S WINS: 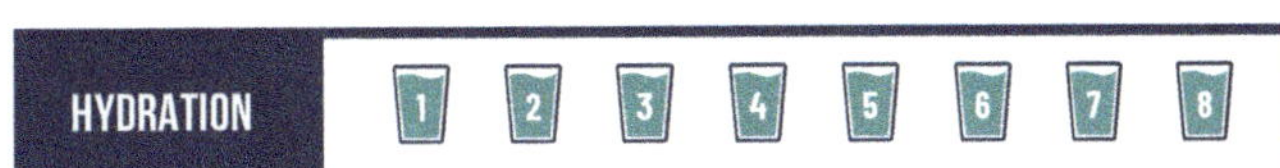

1

2

3

TODAY'S TAKE AWAY:

FOOD FOR THOUGHT FOR THE DAY:

There are more roads than roadblocks.

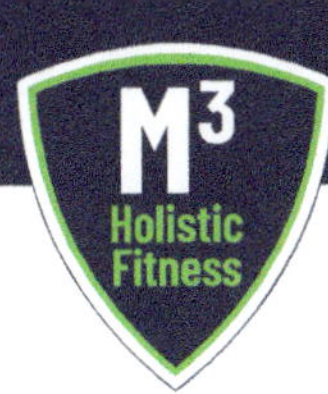

THIS WEEKS WINS:

THIS WEEKS TAKEAWAYS:

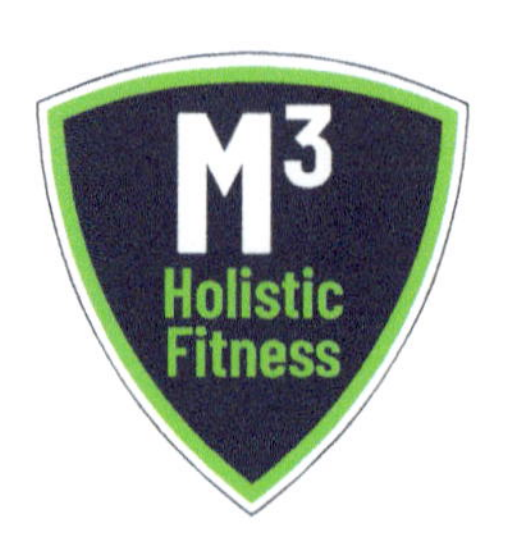

WEEK 4

90-DAY HOLISTIC FITNESS JOURNAL

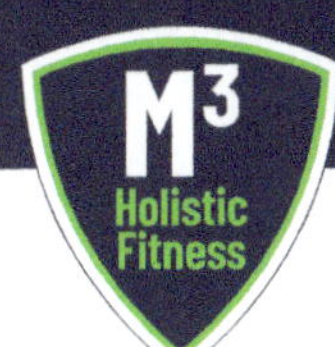

M³ CIRCLE OF LIFE

WHAT DOES YOUR LIFE LOOK LIKE?

1. Place a dot in each category to indicate your level of satisfaction within each area. A dot at the **center of the circle to indicate dissatisfaction,** or towards the **outer edge to indicate satisfaction.** Most people fall somewhere in between. (see example)

2. Connect the dots to see your **M₃ Circle of Life.**

3. Identify imbalances. Determine where to spend more time and energy to create balance. **This will help you create a better balance for your best Badass Life.**

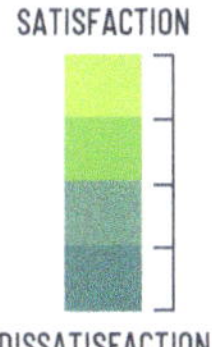

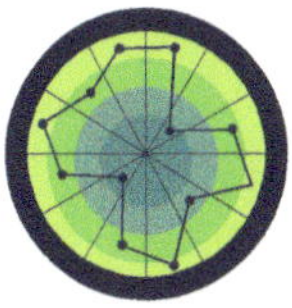

EXAMPLE

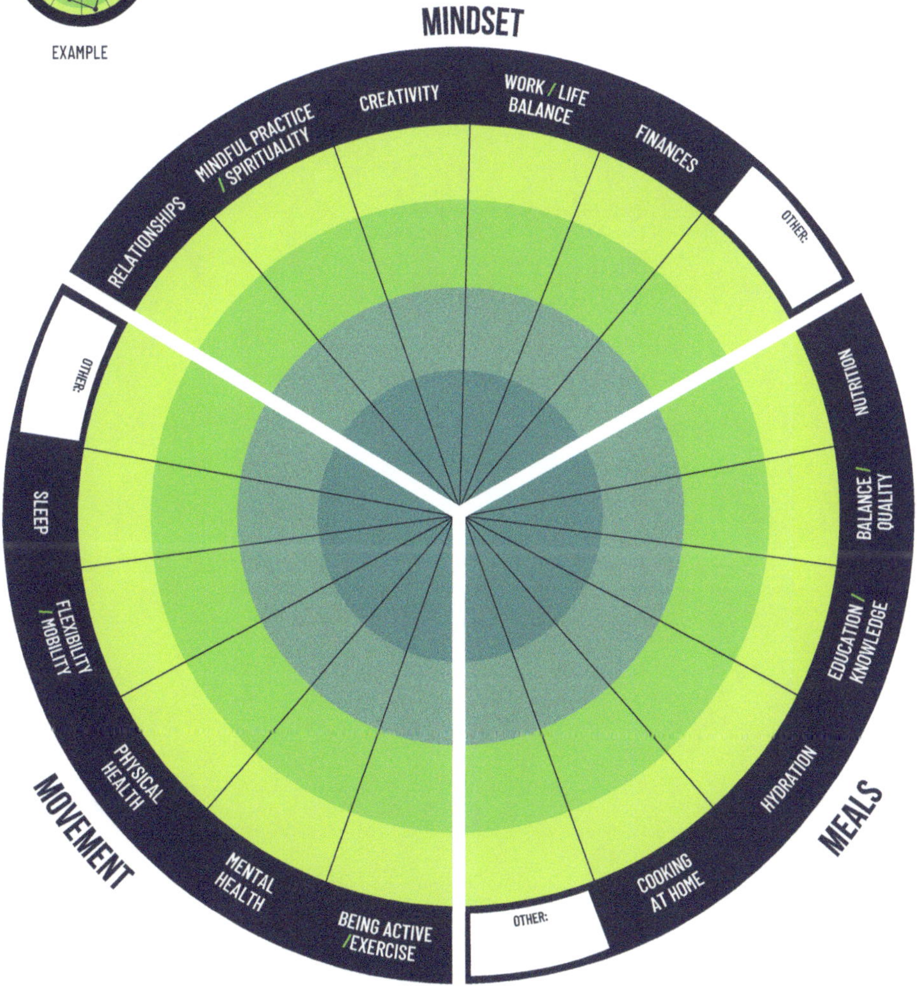

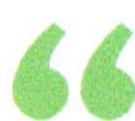

The sky is not the limit.
Your mind is.

- Marilyn Monroe

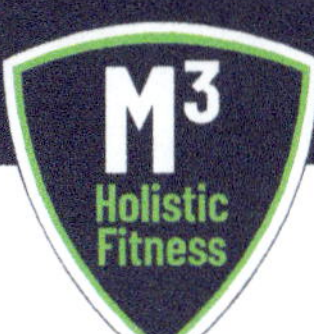

MAKE IT HAPPEN THIS WEEK

 WEEK OF: ____ / ____ / ____

	MINDSET	MOVEMENT	MEALS ✔ ON THE PLATE	MEALS ✔ OFF THE PLATE
MON				
TUES				
WEDS				
THURS				
FRI				
SAT				
SUN				

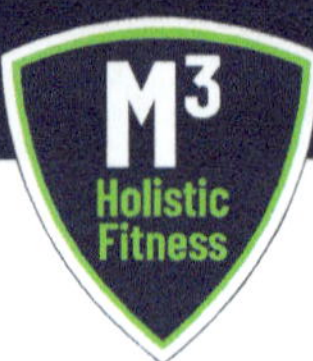

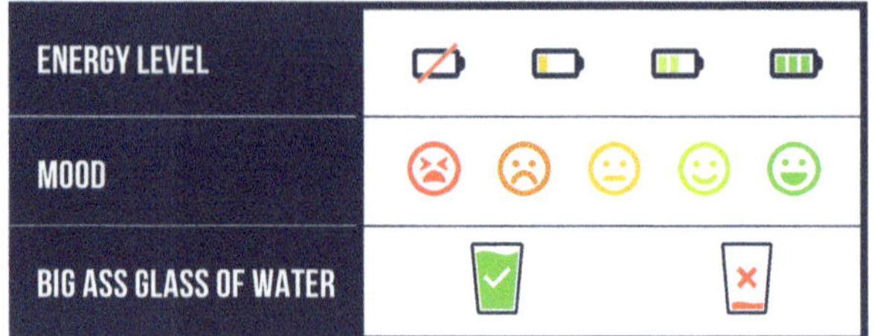

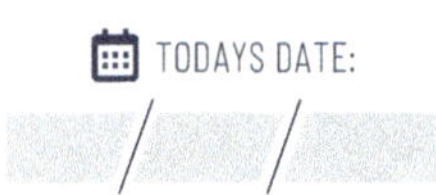

I AM GRATEFUL FOR:

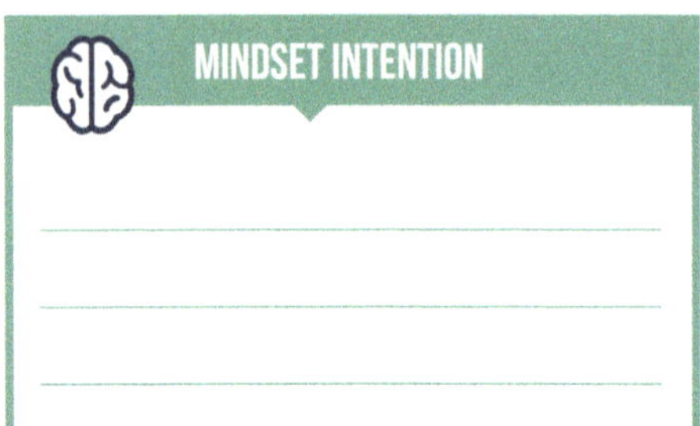

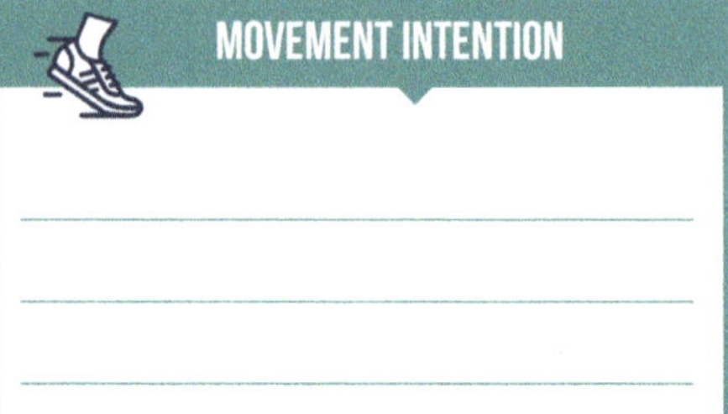

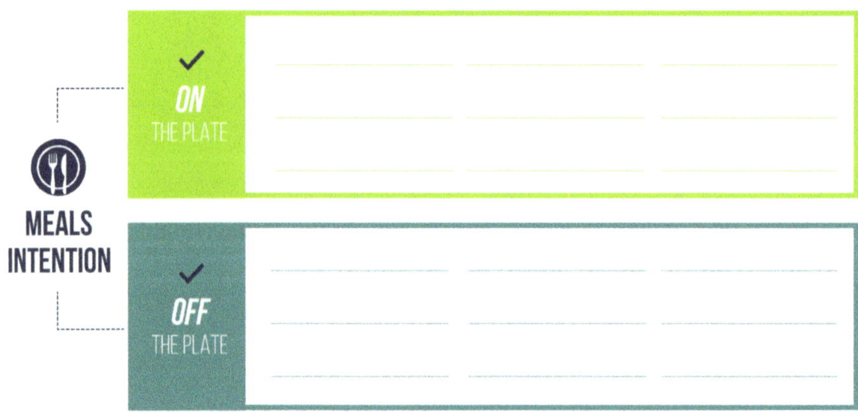

MINDFUL AFFIRMATION:

HYDRATION | 1 | 2 | 3 | 4 | 5 | 6 | 7 | 8

WHAT DIDN'T WORK TODAY?:

MOVEMENT: ☐

MEALS: ☐ ON ☐ OFF

TODAY'S WINS: 

1

2

3

TODAY'S TAKE AWAY:

FOOD FOR THOUGHT FOR THE DAY:

TODAYS DATE: ___/___/___

ENERGY LEVEL				
MOOD				
BIG ASS GLASS OF WATER				

I AM GRATEFUL FOR:

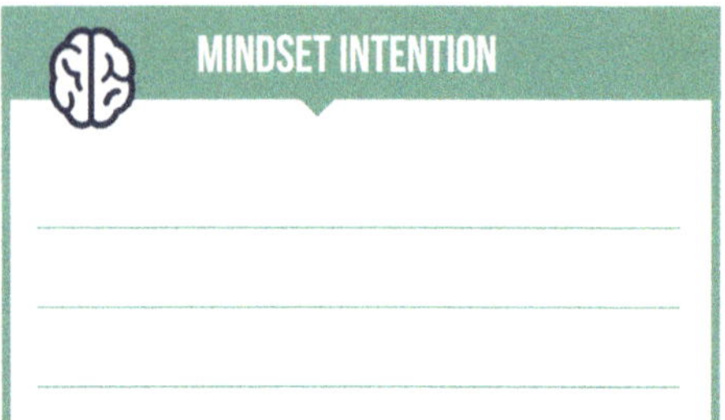

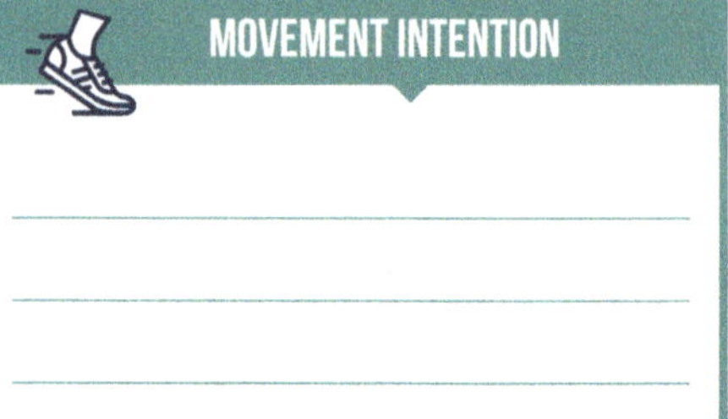

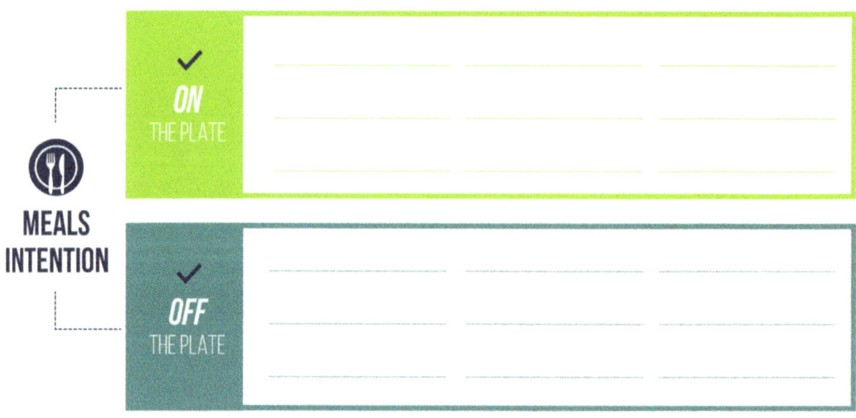

MEALS INTENTION

MINDFUL AFFIRMATION:

WHAT DIDN'T WORK TODAY?:

MOVEMENT: ☐

MEALS: ☐ ON ☐ OFF

TODAY'S WINS: 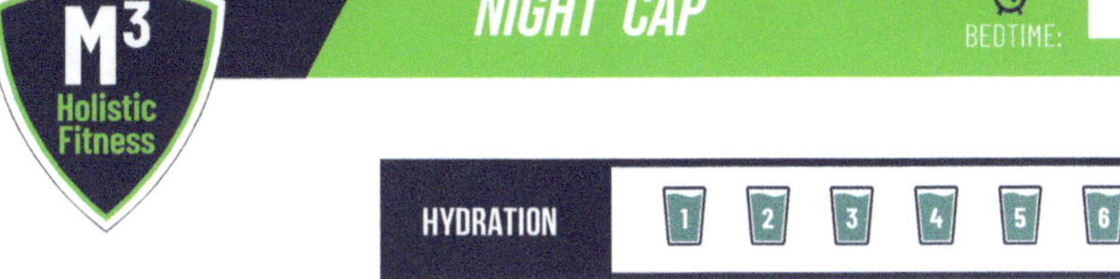

1

2

3

TODAY'S TAKE AWAY:

FOOD FOR THOUGHT FOR THE DAY:

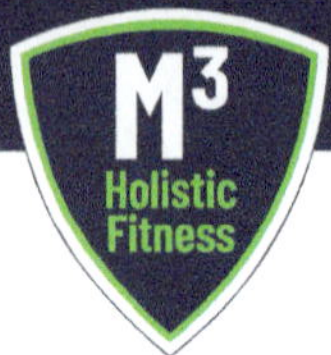

WAKE UP:

SLEEP: Hrs

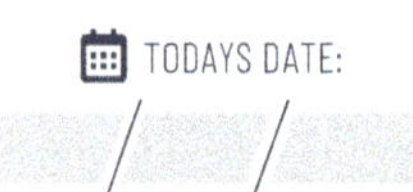

TODAYS DATE:

/ /

ENERGY LEVEL	
MOOD	
BIG ASS GLASS OF WATER	

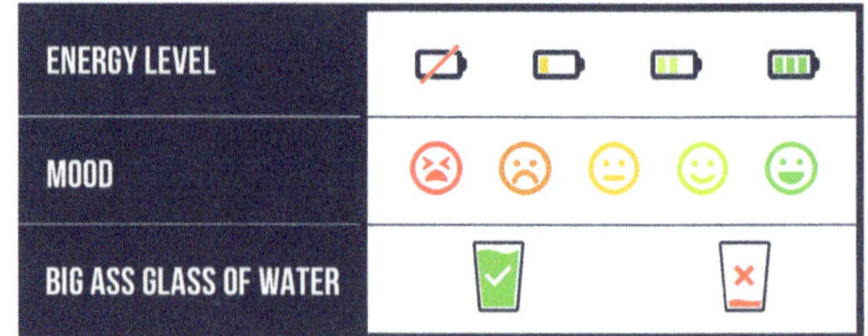

I AM GRATEFUL FOR:

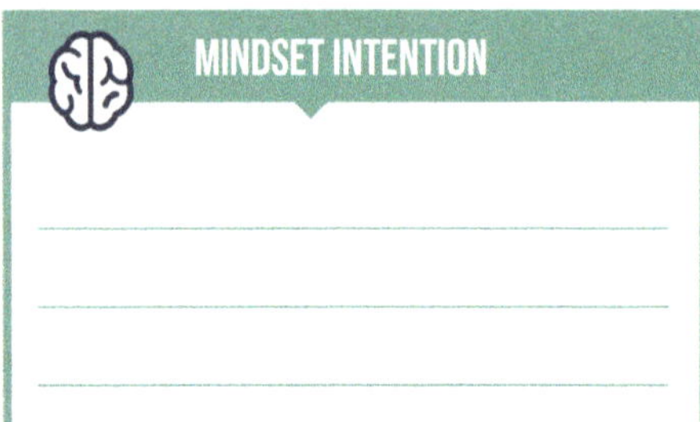

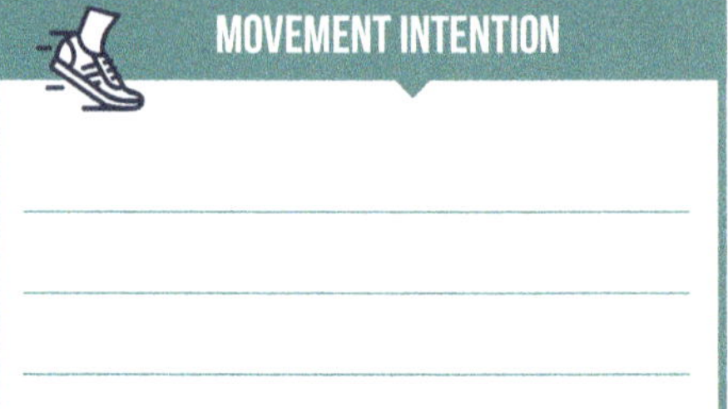

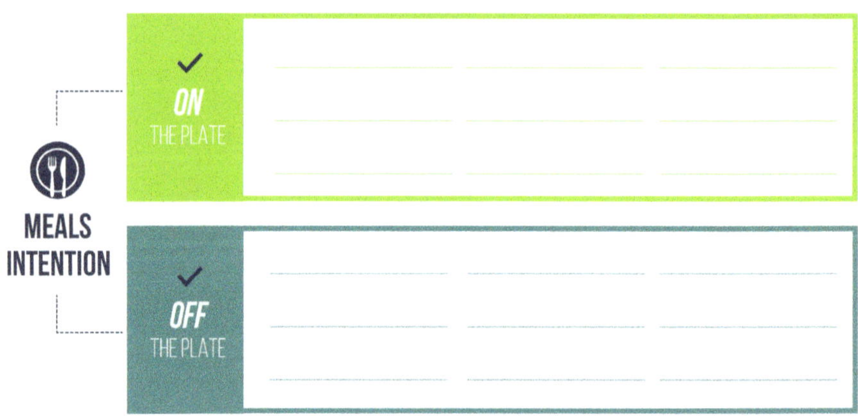

MEALS INTENTION

MINDFUL AFFIRMATION:

HYDRATION   1   2   3   4   5   6   7   8

WHAT DIDN'T WORK TODAY?:

____

MOVEMENT: ☐   MEALS: ☐ ON ☐ OFF

TODAY'S WINS:

1

2

3

TODAY'S TAKE AWAY:

____

FOOD FOR THOUGHT FOR THE DAY:

____

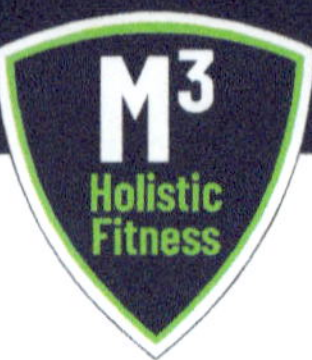

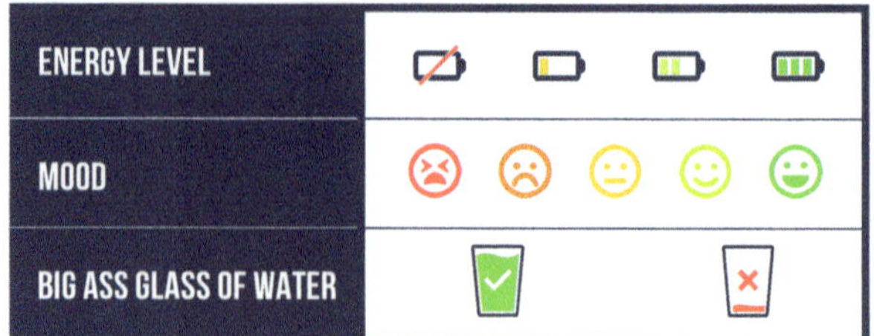

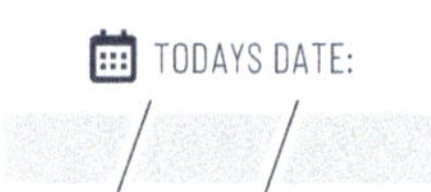

I AM GRATEFUL FOR:

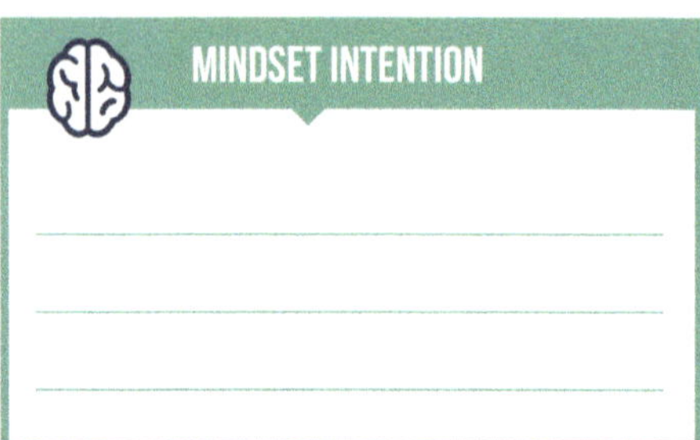

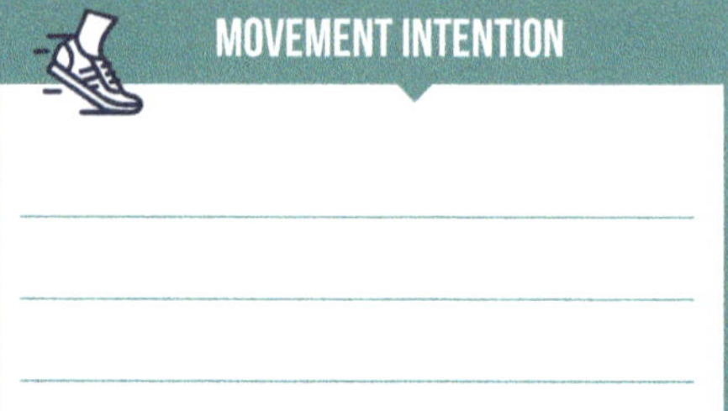

MINDFUL AFFIRMATION:

HYDRATION   1 2 3 4 5 6 7 8

WHAT DIDN'T WORK TODAY?:

MOVEMENT: ☐

MEALS: ☐ ON ☐ OFF

TODAY'S WINS: 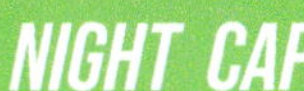

1

2

3

TODAY'S TAKE AWAY:

FOOD FOR THOUGHT FOR THE DAY:

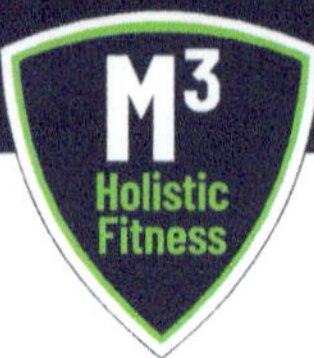

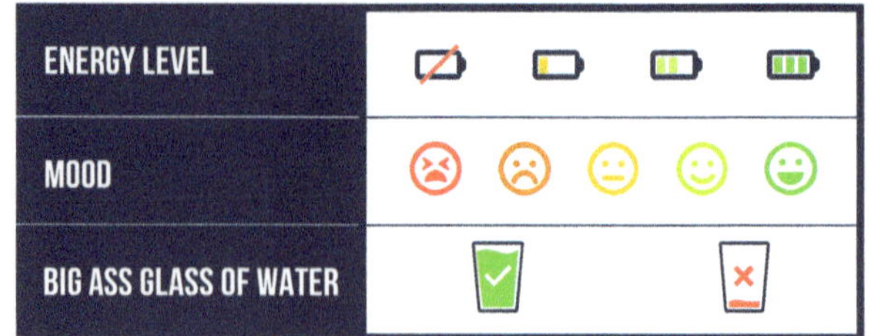

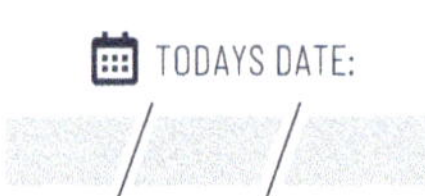

ENERGY LEVEL				
MOOD				
BIG ASS GLASS OF WATER				

I AM GRATEFUL FOR:

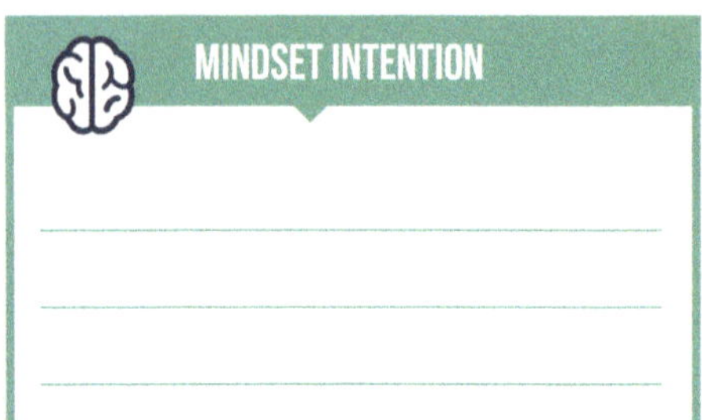

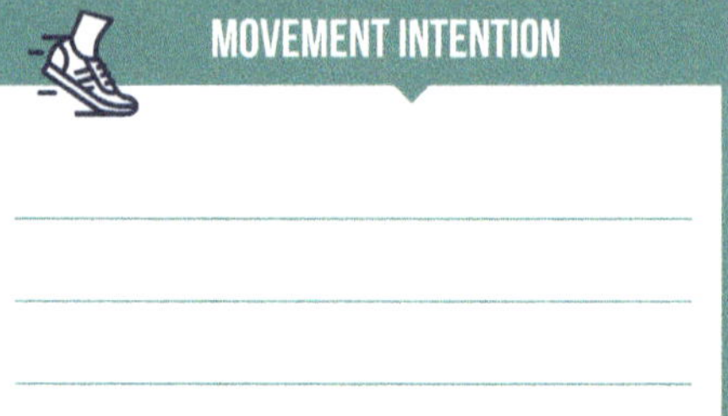

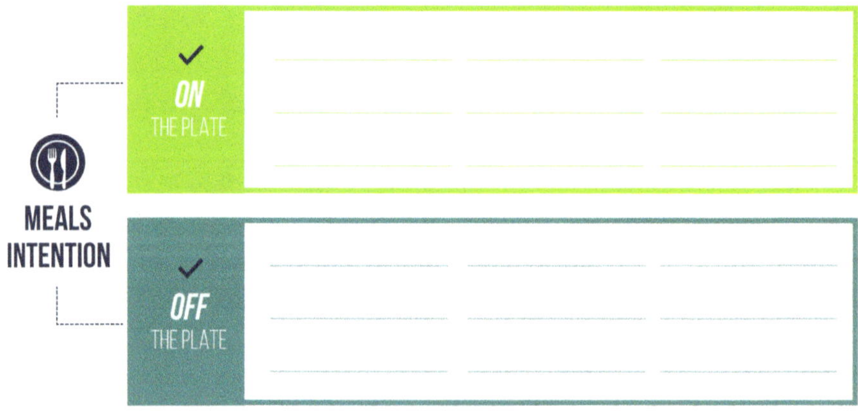

MINDFUL AFFIRMATION:

HYDRATION 1 2 3 4 5 6 7 8

WHAT DIDN'T WORK TODAY?:

____

____

MOVEMENT: ☐

MEALS: ☐ ON   ☐ OFF

TODAY'S WINS: 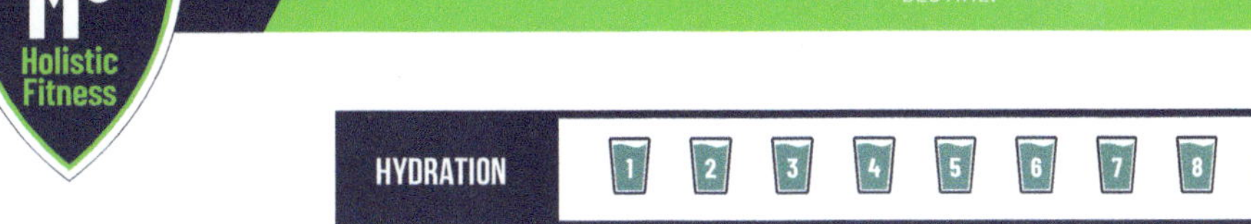

1

2

3

TODAY'S TAKE AWAY:

____

____

____

FOOD FOR THOUGHT FOR THE DAY:

____

____

____

____

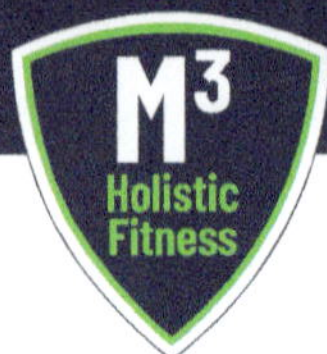

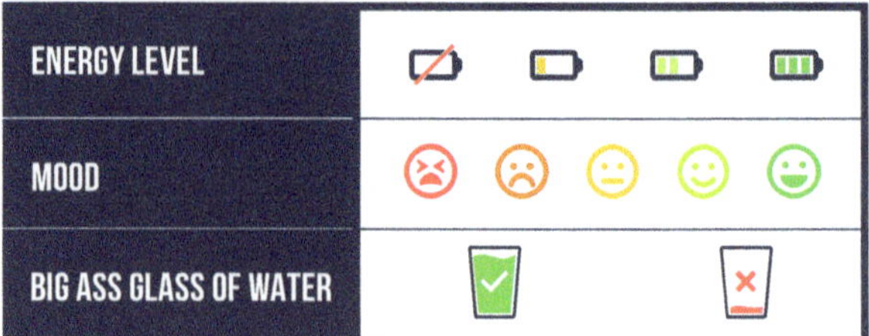

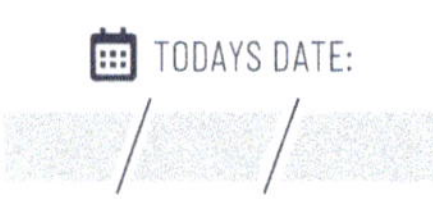

I AM GRATEFUL FOR:

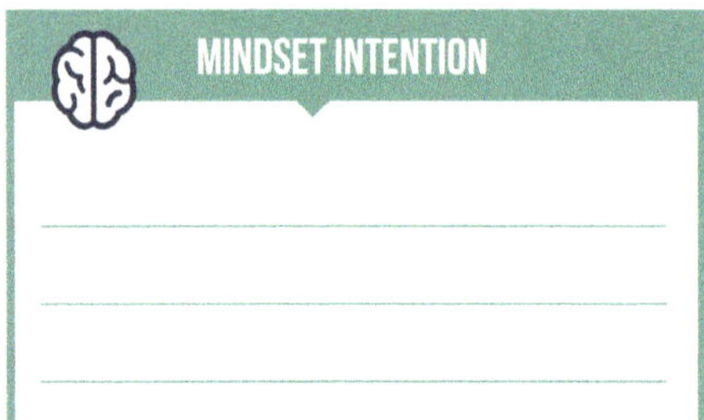

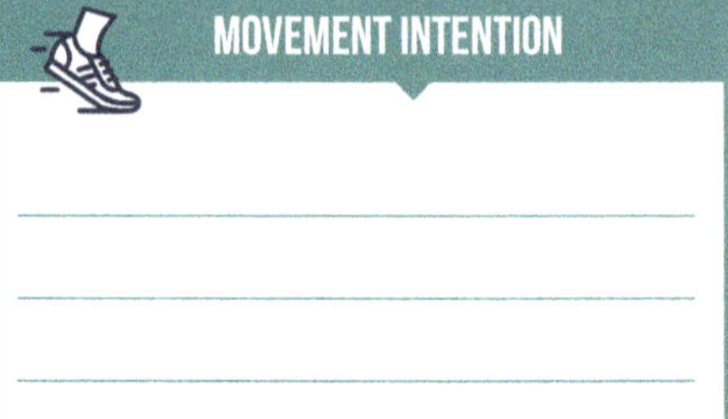

MINDFUL AFFIRMATION:

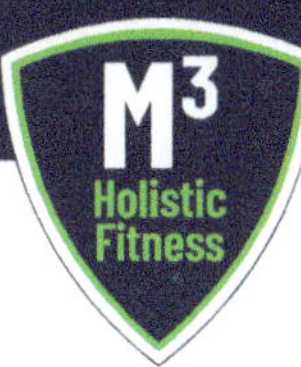

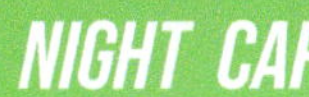

NIGHT CAP

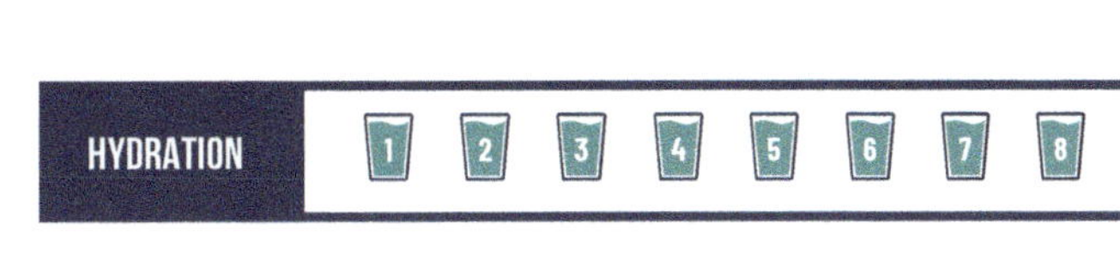

WHAT DIDN'T WORK TODAY?:

MOVEMENT:

MEALS: ON OFF

TODAY'S WINS:

1

2

3

TODAY'S TAKE AWAY:

FOOD FOR THOUGHT FOR THE DAY:

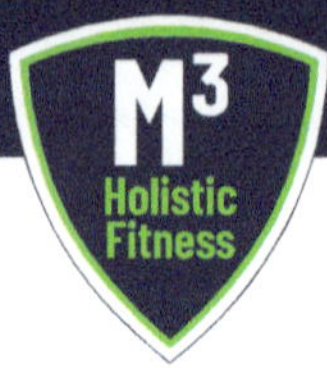

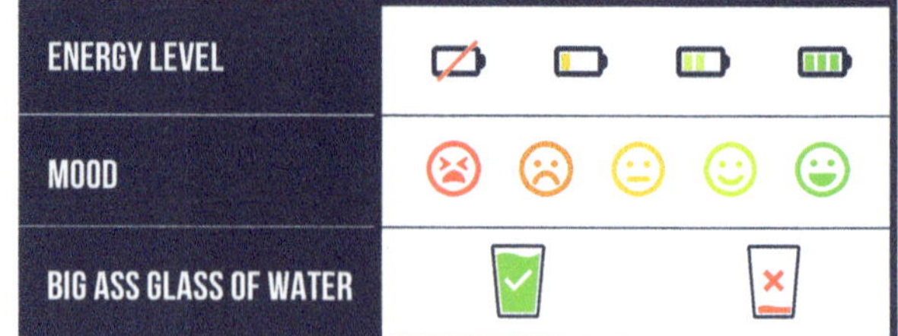

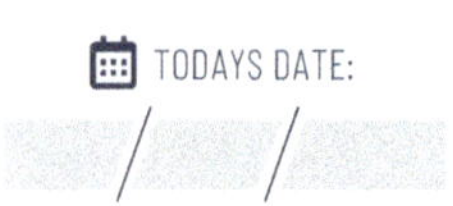

ENERGY LEVEL				
MOOD				
BIG ASS GLASS OF WATER				

I AM GRATEFUL FOR:

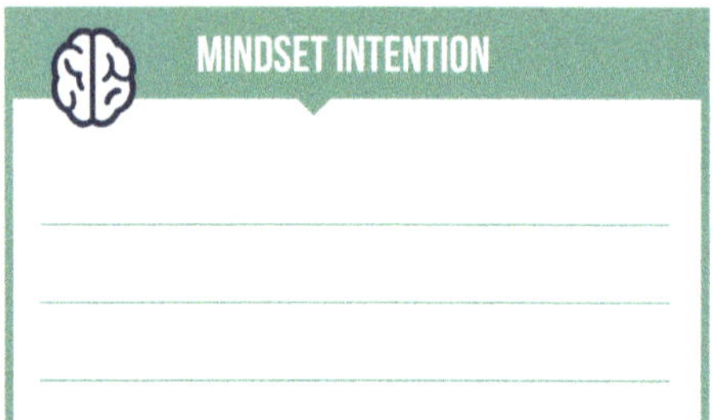

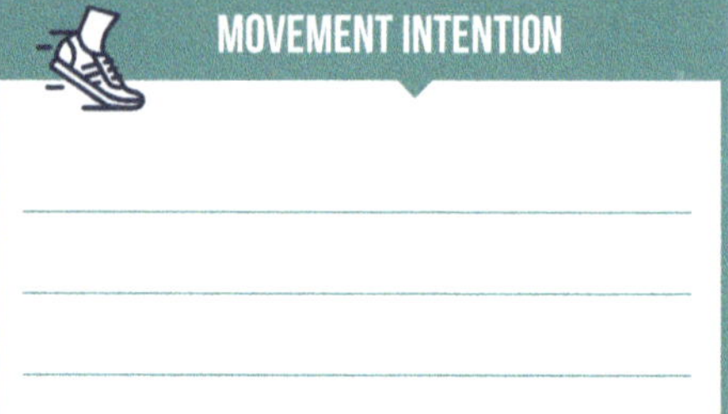

MINDFUL AFFIRMATION:

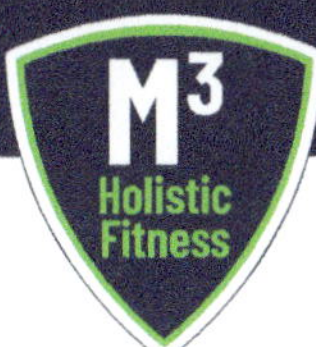

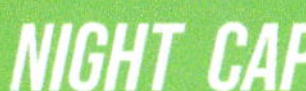

NIGHT CAP

BEDTIME:

HYDRATION 1 2 3 4 5 6 7 8

WHAT DIDN'T WORK TODAY?:

MOVEMENT:

MEALS: ON OFF

TODAY'S WINS:

1

2

3

TODAY'S TAKE AWAY:

FOOD FOR THOUGHT FOR THE DAY:

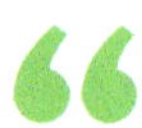

Change is the essence of life. Be willing to sacrifice what you are for what you could become.

- Tony Robbins

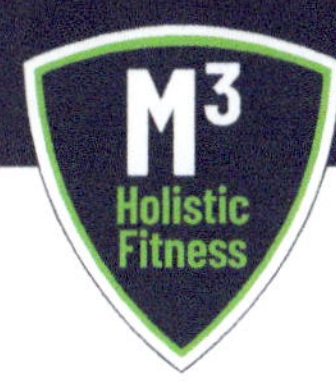

Congratulations on completing your first 30 days of the Rise and Align Journal! You are in the process of creating new habits and becoming a stronger version of yourself. Stay committed to your "WHY"—your vision, your non-negotiables

THE 30 DAYS IN REVIEW:

What are your top 3 wins from the past 30 days?

What have you learned about yourself these past 30 days?

What are the M3 outcomes you want out of the next 30 days?

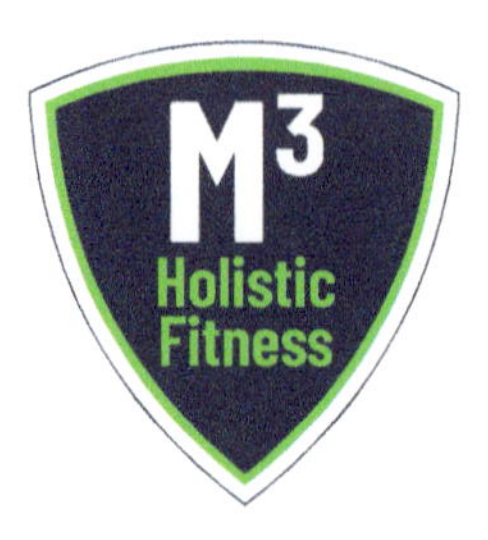

WEEK 5

90-DAY HOLISTIC FITNESS JOURNAL

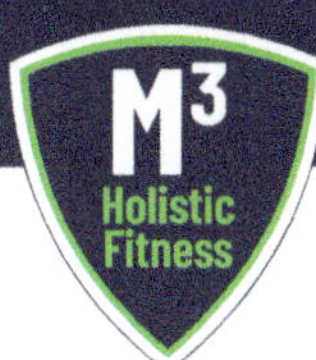

WHAT DOES YOUR LIFE LOOK LIKE?

1. Place a dot in each category to indicate your level of satisfaction within each area. A dot at the **center of the circle to indicate dissatisfaction**, or towards the **outer edge to indicate satisfaction**. Most people fall somewhere in between. (see example)

2. Connect the dots to see your M3 **Circle of Life.**

3. Identify imbalances. Determine where to spend more time and energy to create balance. **This will help you create a better balance for your best Badass Life.**

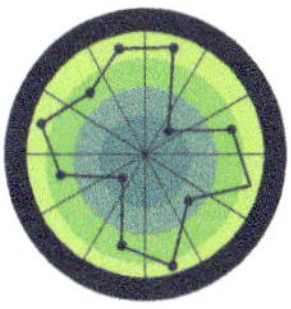

SATISFACTION

DISSATISFACTION

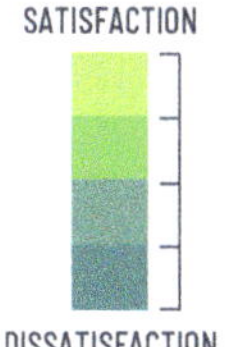

EXAMPLE

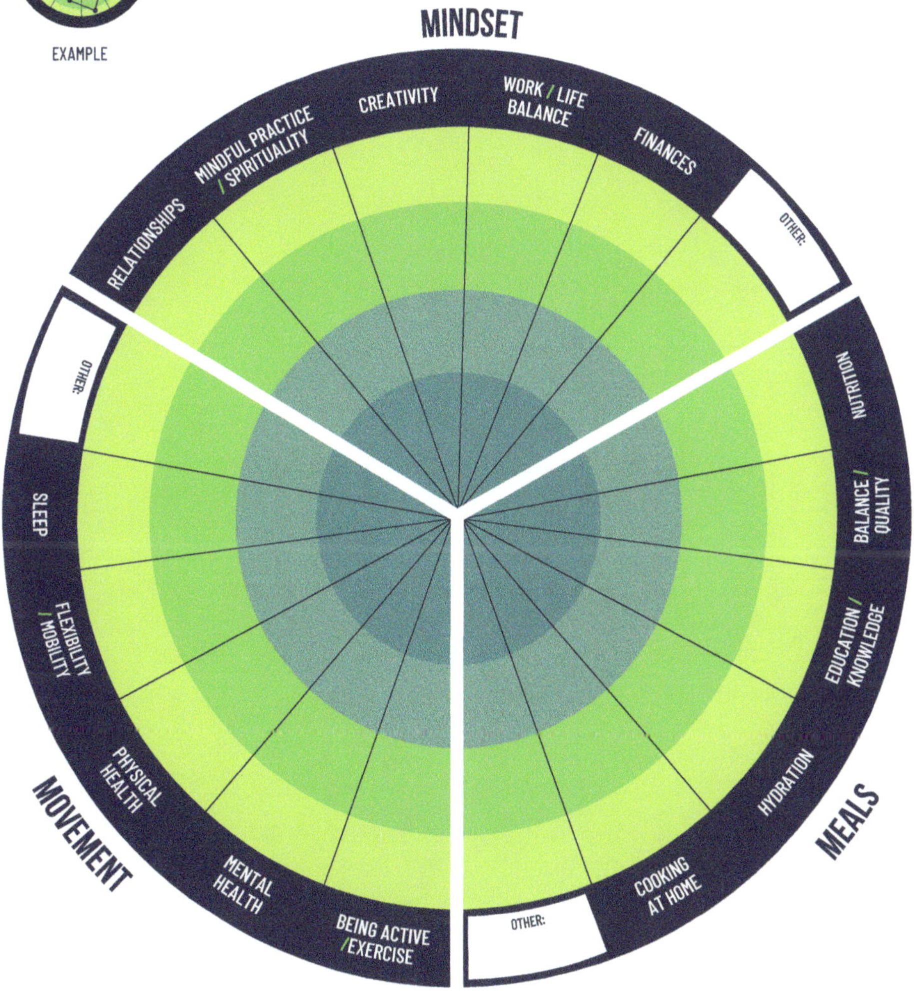

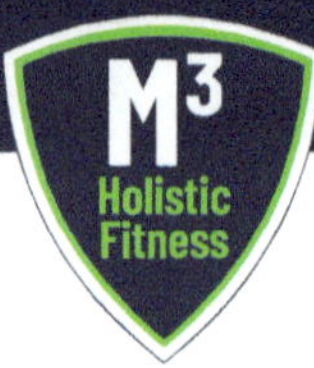

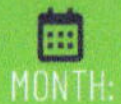

MONTH:

HABIT

DAY							
1							
2							
3							
4							
5							
6							
7							
8							
9							
10							
11							
12							
13							
14							
15							
16							
17							
18							
19							
20							
21							
22							
23							
24							
25							
26							
27							
28							
29							
30							
31							
TOTAL							

M3 Holistic Fitness

MAKE IT HAPPEN THIS WEEK

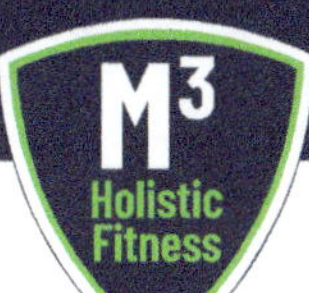

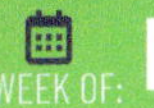

WEEK OF: __/__/__

	MINDSET	MOVEMENT	MEALS ✓ ON THE PLATE	✓ OFF THE PLATE
MON				
TUES				
WEDS				
THURS				
FRI				
SAT				
SUN				

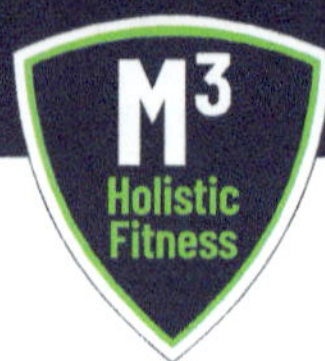

RISE AND ALIGN

WAKE UP: SLEEP: Hrs

ENERGY LEVEL				
MOOD				
BIG ASS GLASS OF WATER				

TODAYS DATE: ___ / ___ / ___

I AM GRATEFUL FOR:

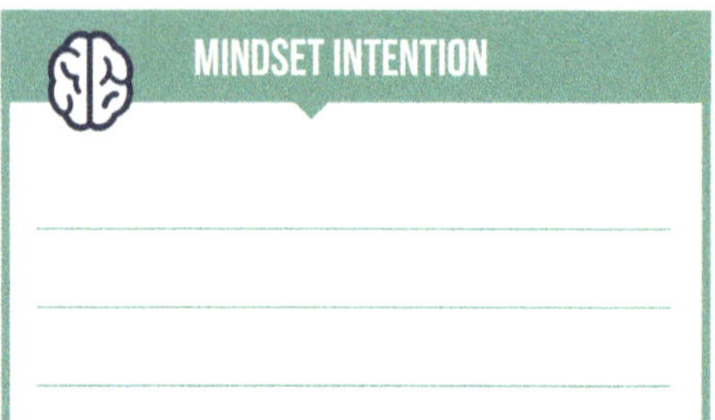

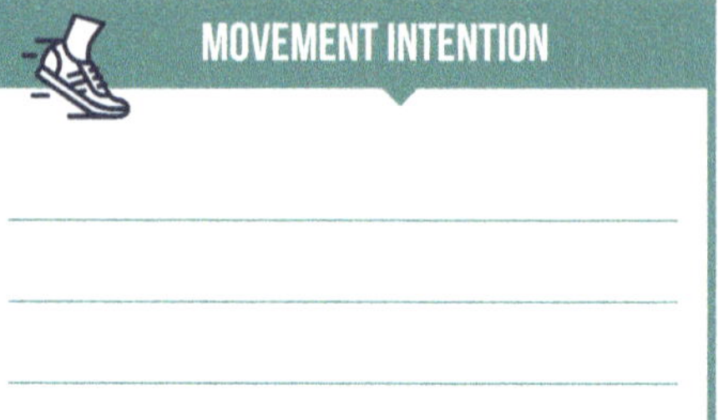

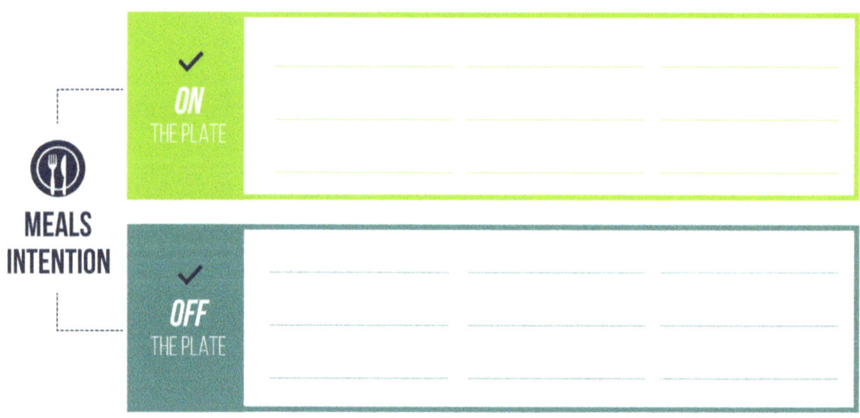

MINDFUL AFFIRMATION:

HYDRATION | 1 | 2 | 3 | 4 | 5 | 6 | 7 | 8

WHAT DIDN'T WORK TODAY?:

MOVEMENT: ☐

MEALS: ☐ ON ☐ OFF

TODAY'S WINS: 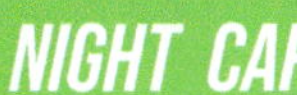

1

2

3

TODAY'S TAKE AWAY:

FOOD FOR THOUGHT FOR THE DAY:

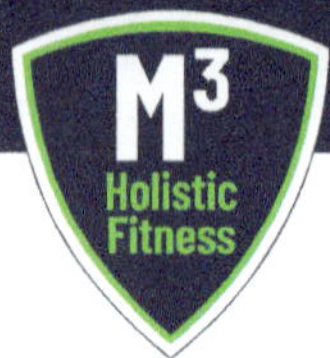

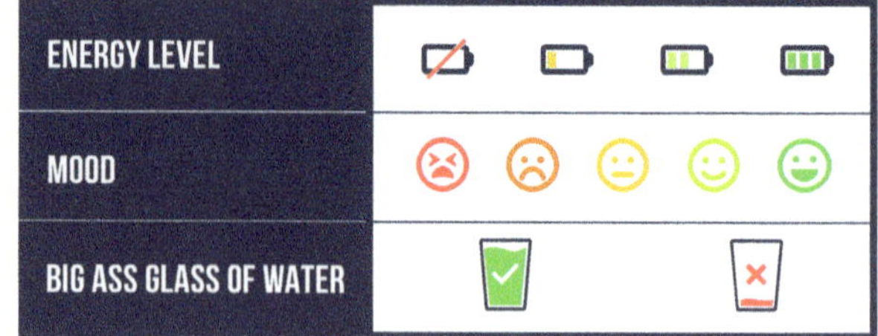

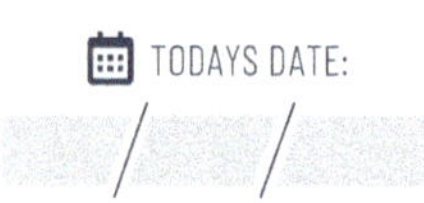

ENERGY LEVEL				
MOOD				
BIG ASS GLASS OF WATER				

I AM GRATEFUL FOR:

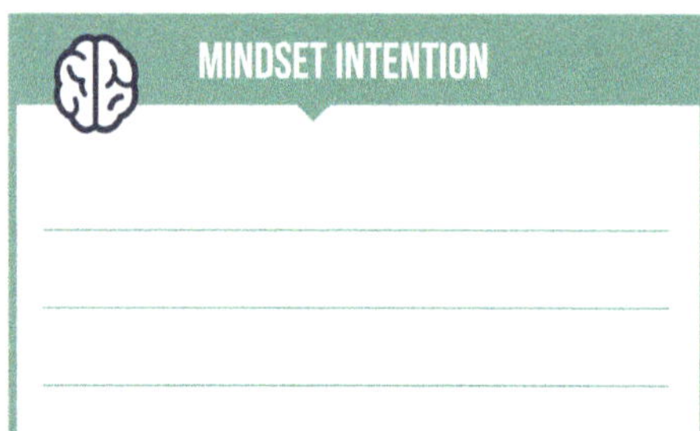

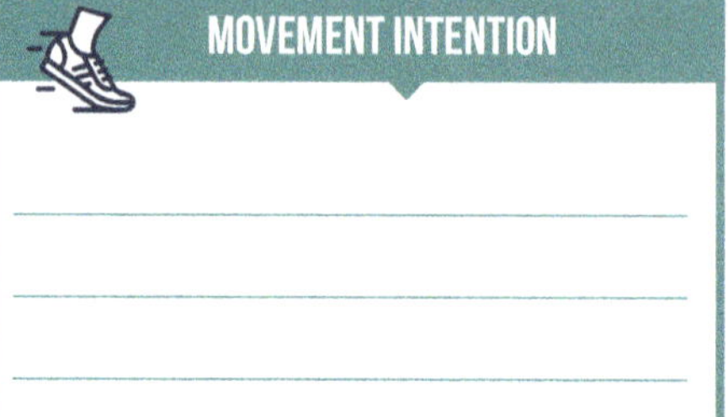

MINDFUL AFFIRMATION:

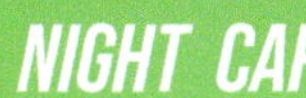
NIGHT CAP

BEDTIME:

HYDRATION | 1 | 2 | 3 | 4 | 5 | 6 | 7 | 8 |

WHAT DIDN'T WORK TODAY?:

MOVEMENT: ☐

MEALS: ☐ ON ☐ OFF

TODAY'S WINS:

1

2

3

TODAY'S TAKE AWAY:

FOOD FOR THOUGHT FOR THE DAY:

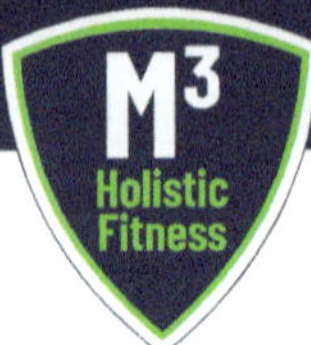

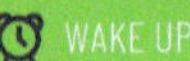
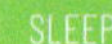

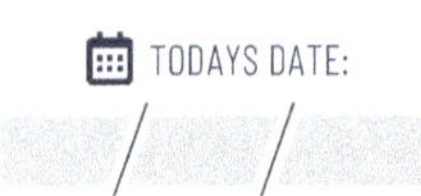

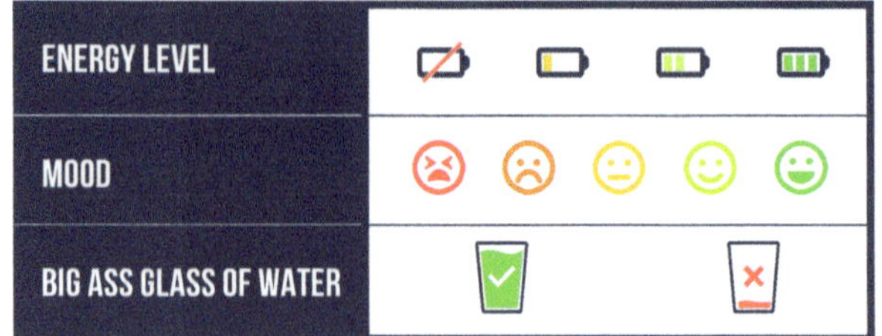

I AM GRATEFUL FOR:

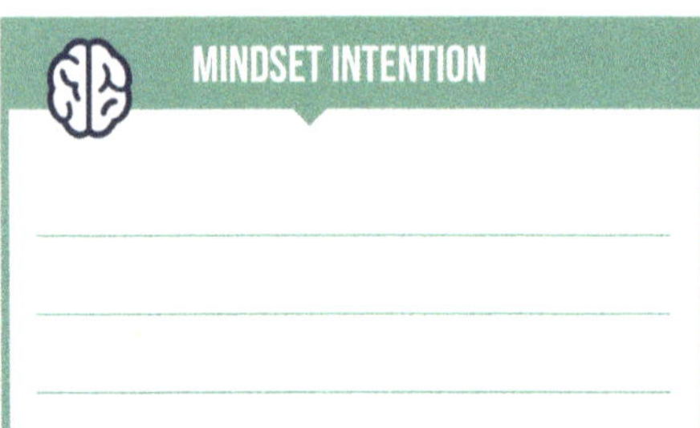

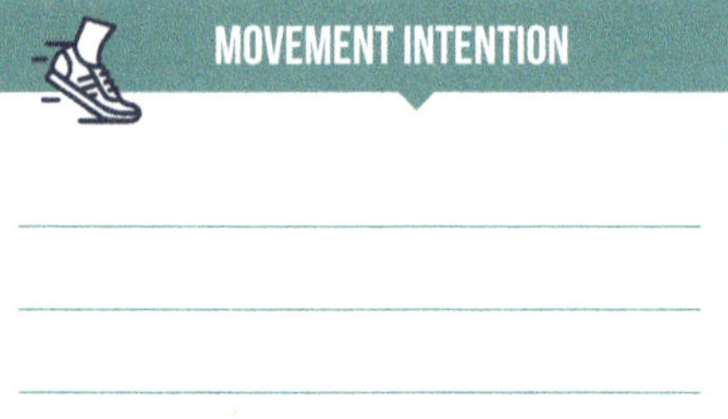

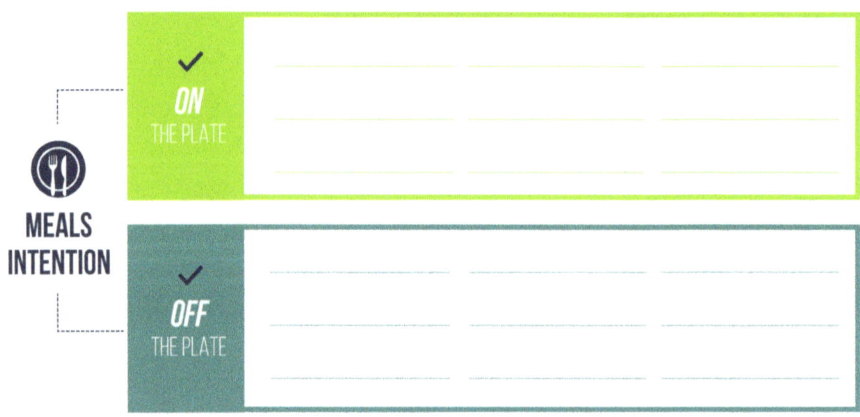

MINDFUL AFFIRMATION:

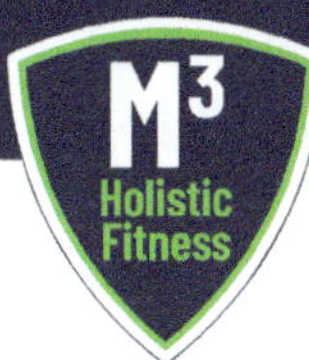

NIGHT CAP

BEDTIME:

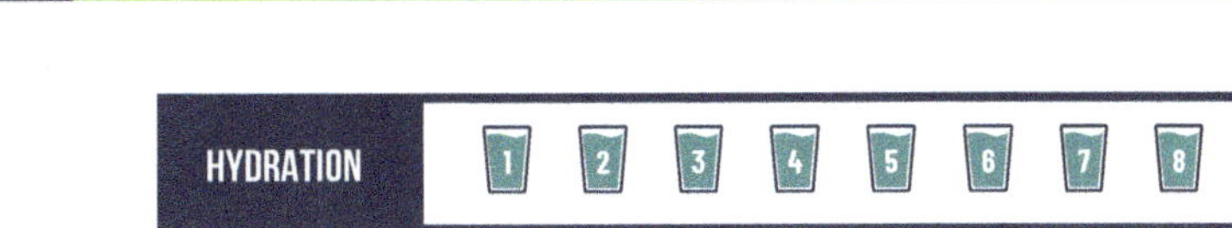

WHAT DIDN'T WORK TODAY?:

MOVEMENT: ☐

MEALS: ☐ ON ☐ OFF

TODAY'S WINS: 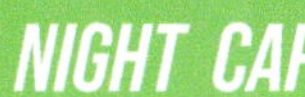

1

2

3

TODAY'S TAKE AWAY:

FOOD FOR THOUGHT FOR THE DAY:

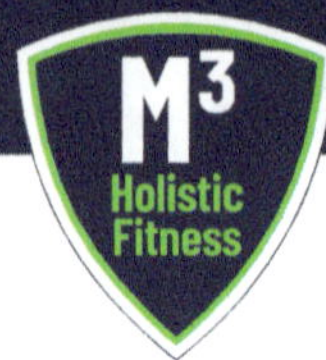

WAKE UP: | SLEEP: Hrs

ENERGY LEVEL				
MOOD				
BIG ASS GLASS OF WATER				

TODAYS DATE: ___ / ___ / ___

I AM GRATEFUL FOR:

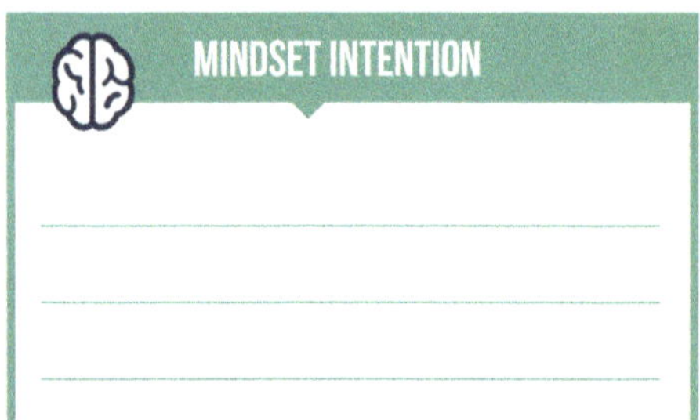

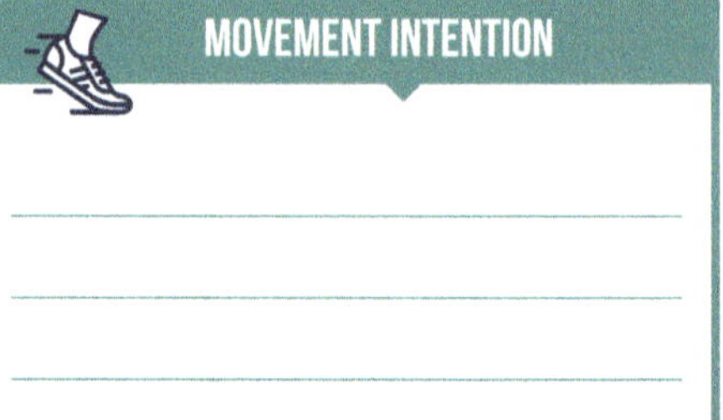

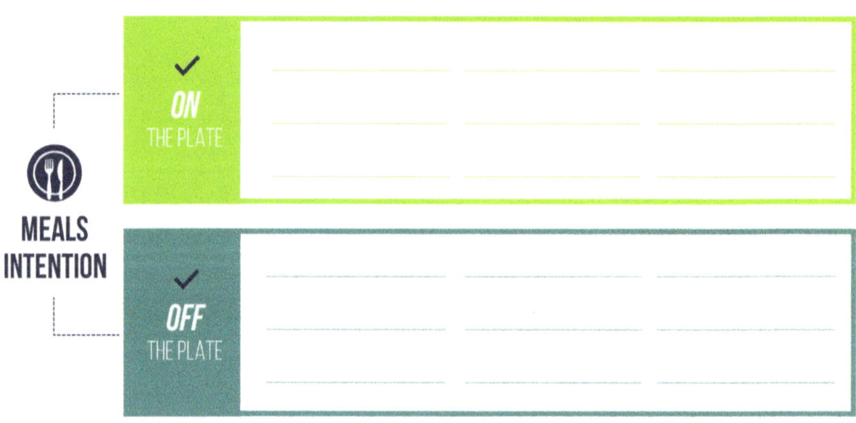

MEALS INTENTION

MINDFUL AFFIRMATION:

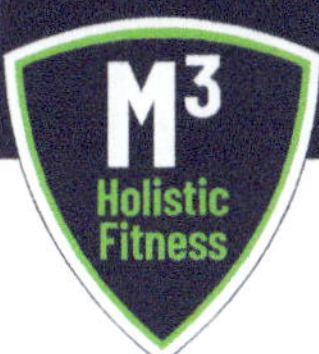

NIGHT CAP

BEDTIME:

HYDRATION | 1 | 2 | 3 | 4 | 5 | 6 | 7 | 8 |

WHAT DIDN'T WORK TODAY?:

MOVEMENT: ☐

MEALS: ☐ ON ☐ OFF

TODAY'S WINS: 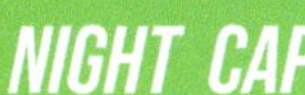

1

2

3

TODAY'S TAKE AWAY:

FOOD FOR THOUGHT FOR THE DAY:

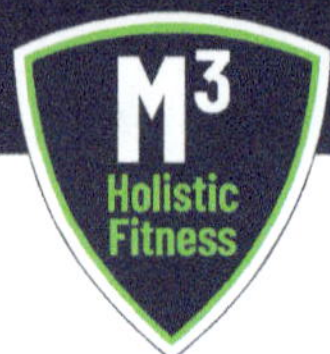

ENERGY LEVEL				
MOOD				
BIG ASS GLASS OF WATER				

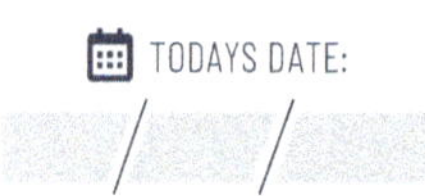 TODAYS DATE:

___ / ___ / ___

I AM GRATEFUL FOR:

MINDSET INTENTION

MOVEMENT INTENTION

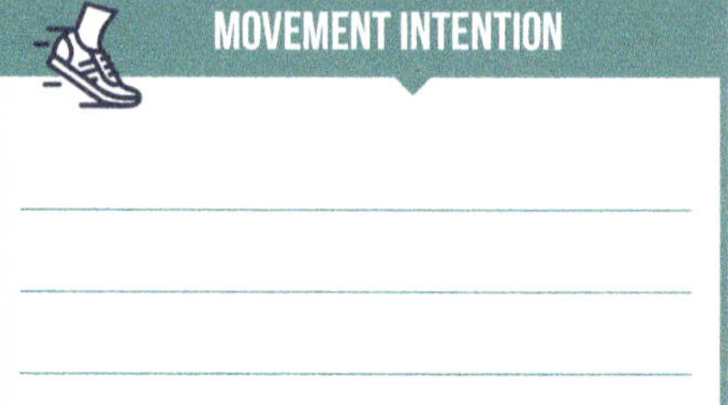

MEALS INTENTION

ON THE PLATE

OFF THE PLATE

MINDFUL AFFIRMATION:

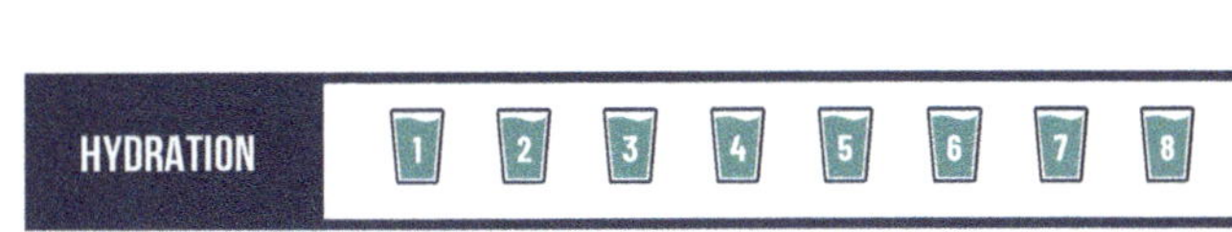

WHAT DIDN'T WORK TODAY?:

MOVEMENT:

MEALS: ON OFF

TODAY'S WINS: 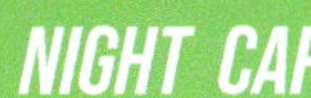

1

2

3

TODAY'S TAKE AWAY:

FOOD FOR THOUGHT FOR THE DAY:

Holistic Fitness

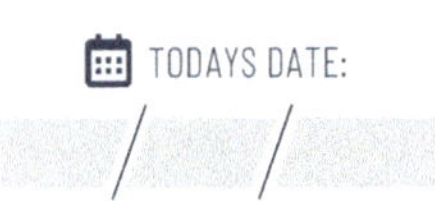

ENERGY LEVEL				
MOOD				
BIG ASS GLASS OF WATER				

I AM GRATEFUL FOR:

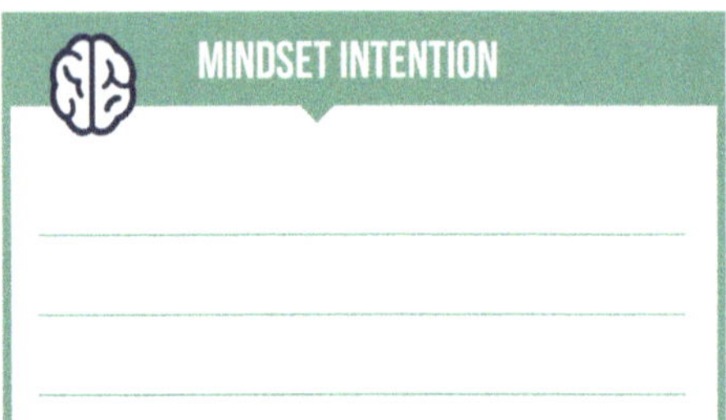

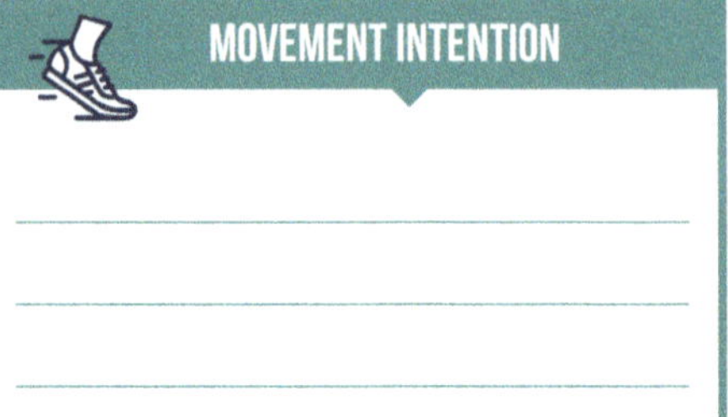

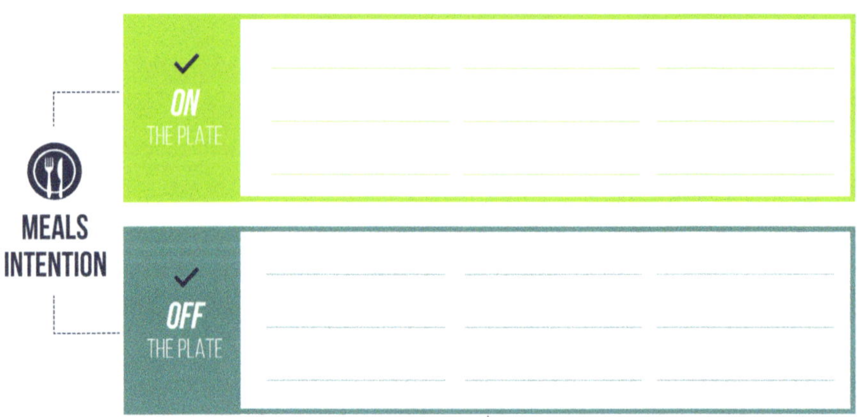

MEALS INTENTION

MINDFUL AFFIRMATION:

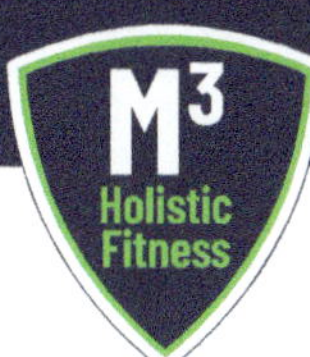

NIGHT CAP

HYDRATION 1 2 3 4 5 6 7 8

WHAT DIDN'T WORK TODAY?:

MOVEMENT: ☐

MEALS: ☐ ON ☐ OFF

TODAY'S WINS:

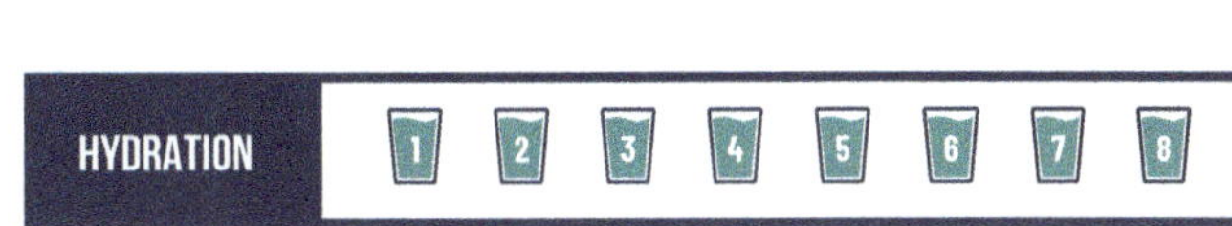

1

2

3

TODAY'S TAKE AWAY:

FOOD FOR THOUGHT FOR THE DAY:

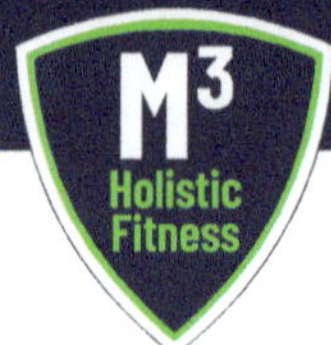

ENERGY LEVEL				
MOOD				
BIG ASS GLASS OF WATER				

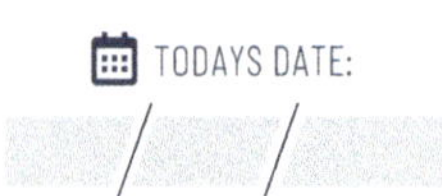 TODAYS DATE: _____ / _____ / _____

I AM GRATEFUL FOR:

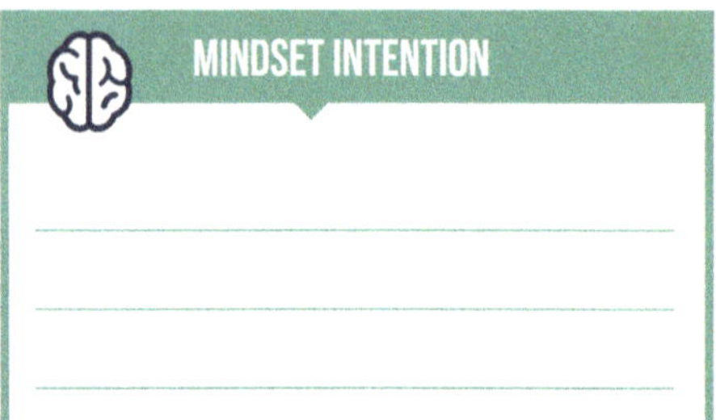

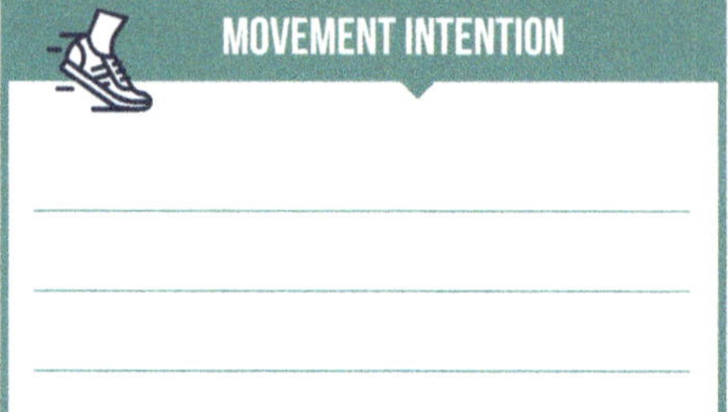

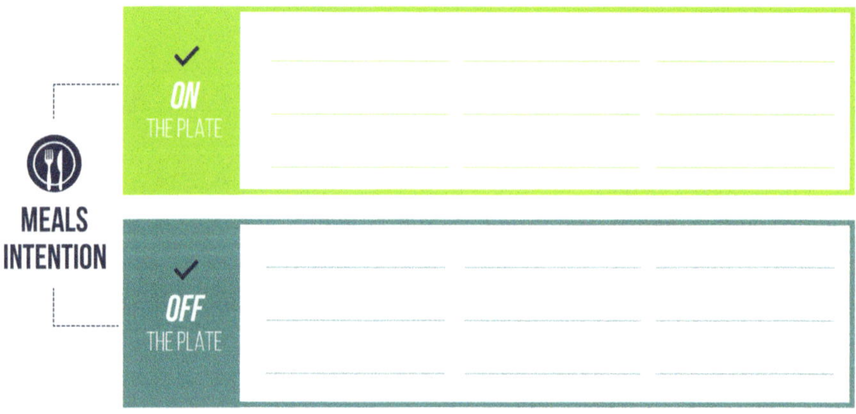

MINDFUL AFFIRMATION:

HYDRATION 1 2 3 4 5 6 7 8

WHAT DIDN'T WORK TODAY?:

MOVEMENT: ☐

MEALS: ☐ ON ☐ OFF

TODAY'S WINS:

1

2

3

TODAY'S TAKE AWAY:

FOOD FOR THOUGHT FOR THE DAY:

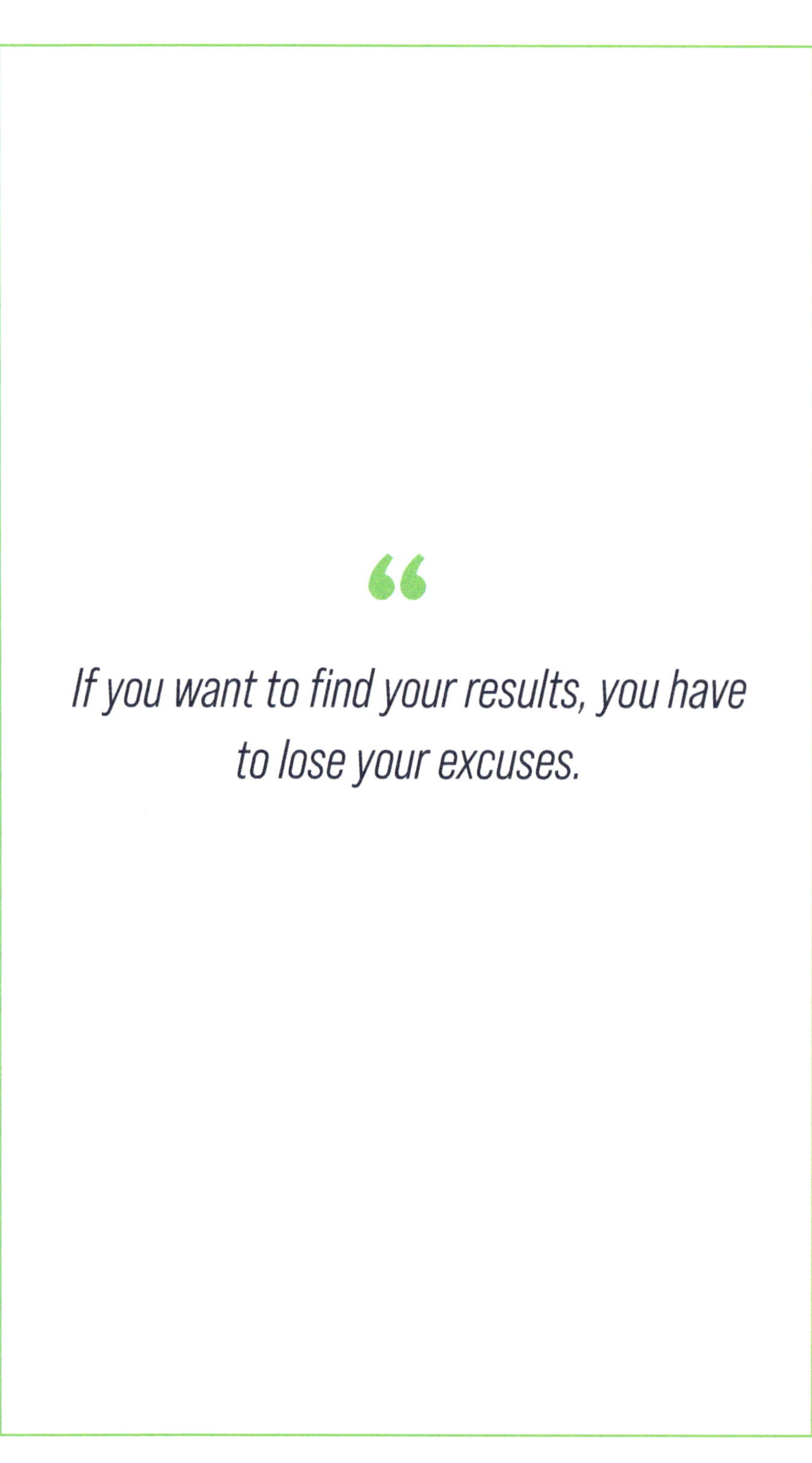

If you want to find your results, you have to lose your excuses.

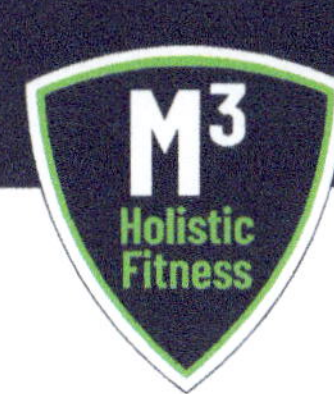

THIS WEEKS WINS:

THIS WEEKS TAKEAWAYS:

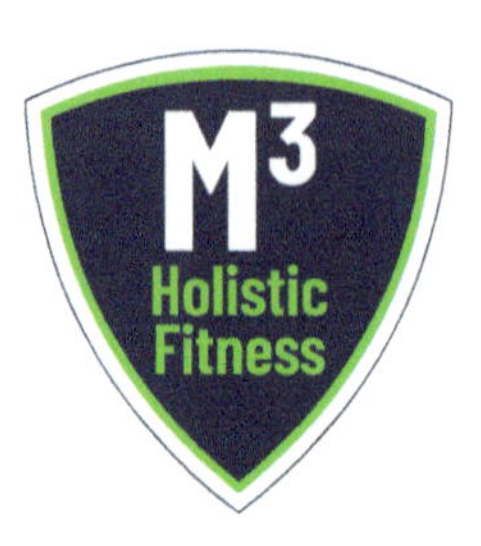

WEEK 6

90-DAY HOLISTIC FITNESS JOURNAL

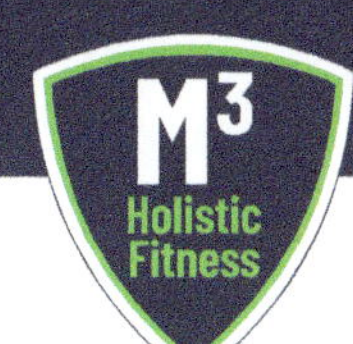

WHAT DOES YOUR LIFE LOOK LIKE?

SATISFACTION

DISSATISFACTION

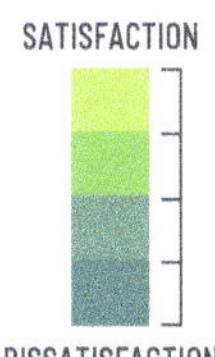

EXAMPLE

1. Place a dot in each category to indicate your level of satisfaction within each area. A dot at the **center of the circle to indicate dissatisfaction**, or towards the **outer edge to indicate satisfaction**. Most people fall somewhere in between. (see example)

2. Connect the dots to see your M3 **Circle of Life**.

3. Identify imbalances. Determine where to spend more time and energy to create balance. **This will help you create a better balance for your best Badass Life.**

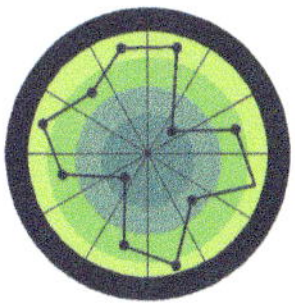

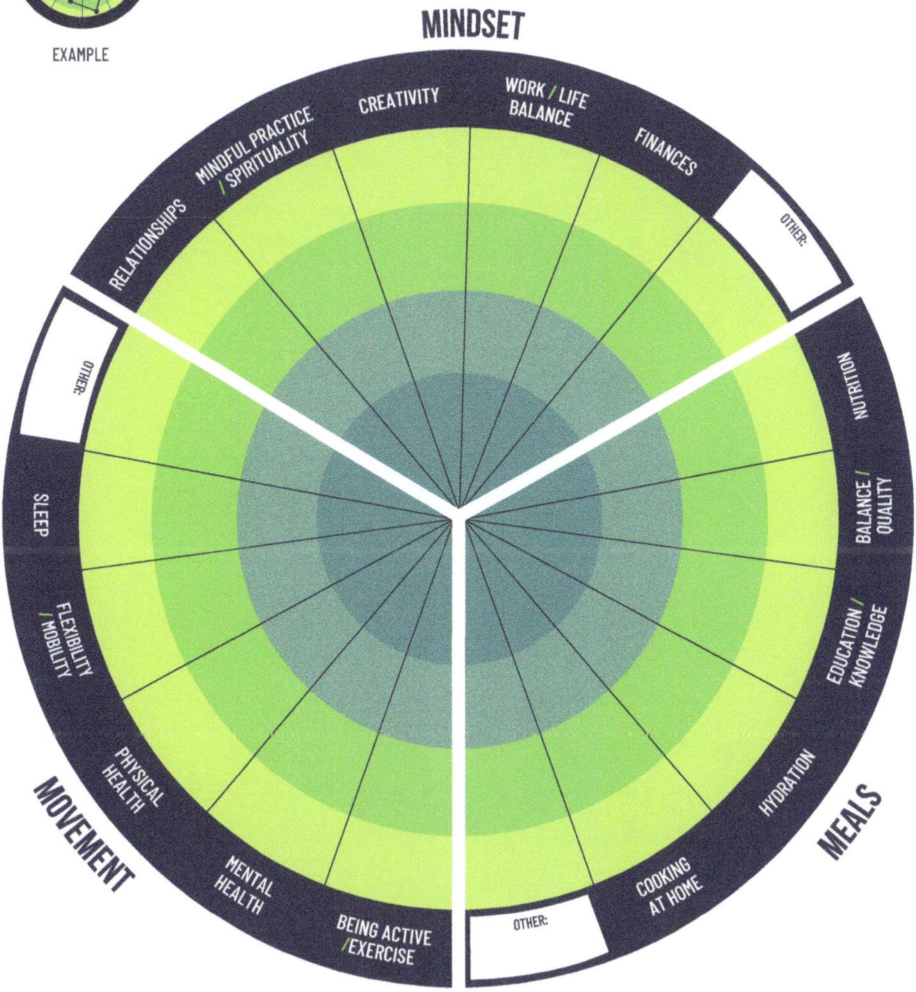

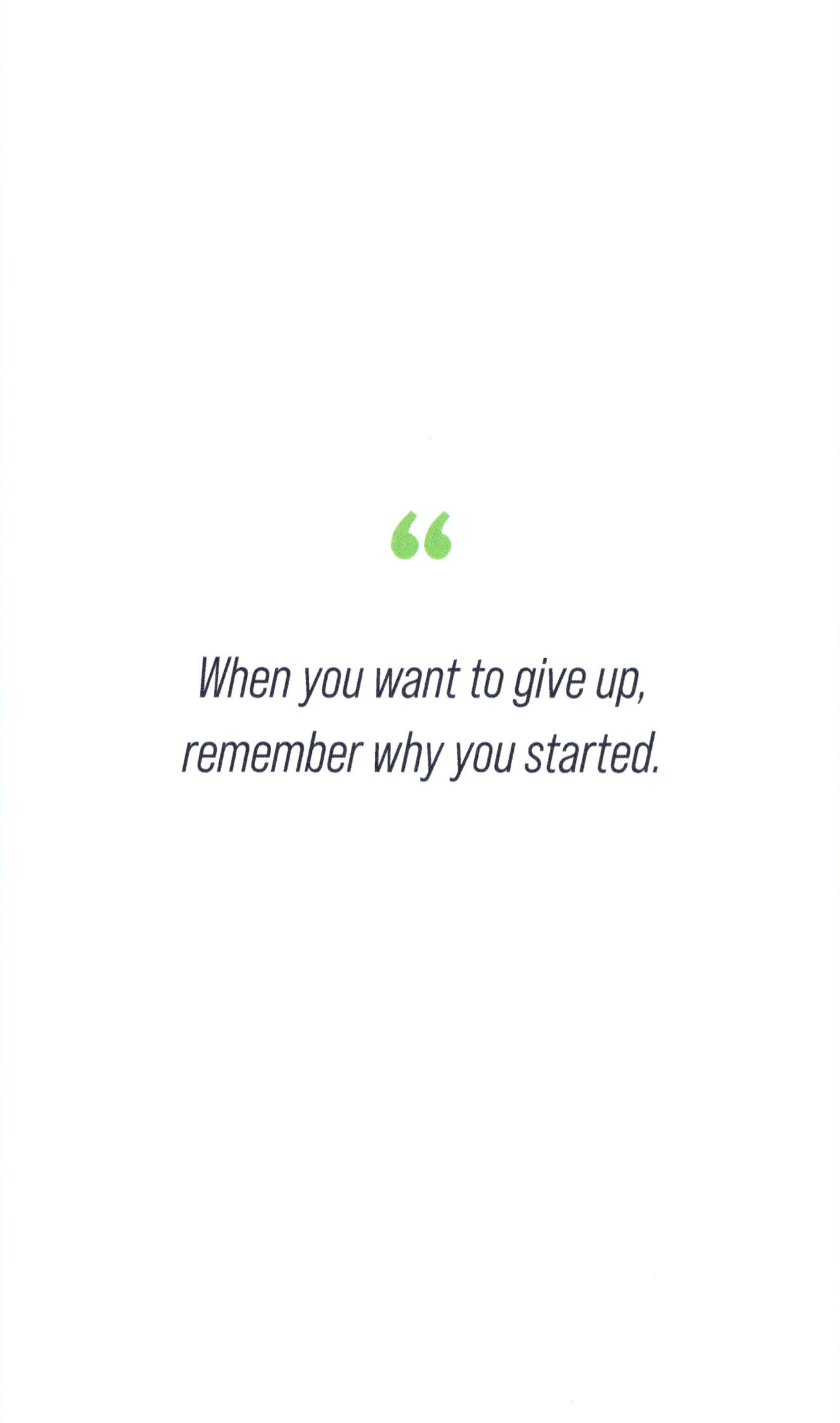

When you want to give up,
remember why you started.

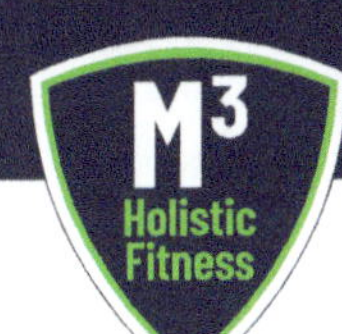

	MINDSET	MOVEMENT	MEALS ✓ ON THE PLATE	✓ OFF THE PLATE
MON				
TUES				
WEDS				
THURS				
FRI				
SAT				
SUN				

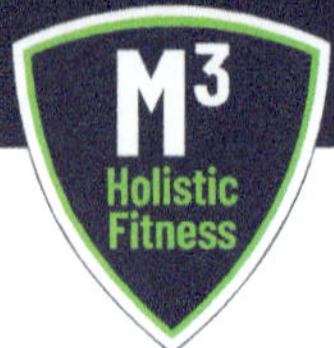

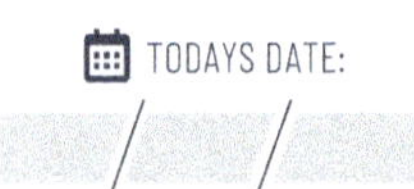

ENERGY LEVEL				
MOOD				
BIG ASS GLASS OF WATER				

I AM GRATEFUL FOR:

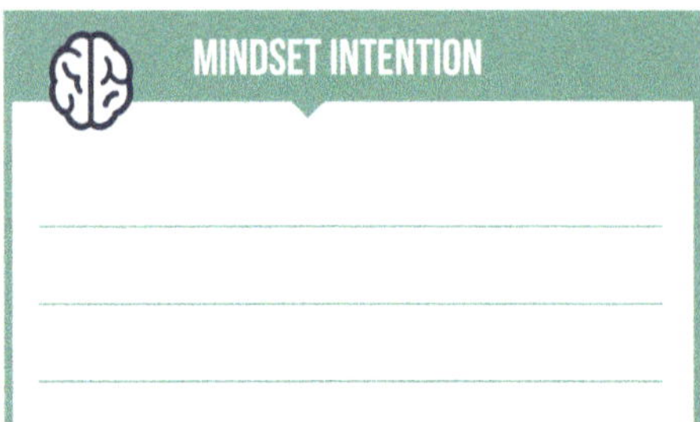

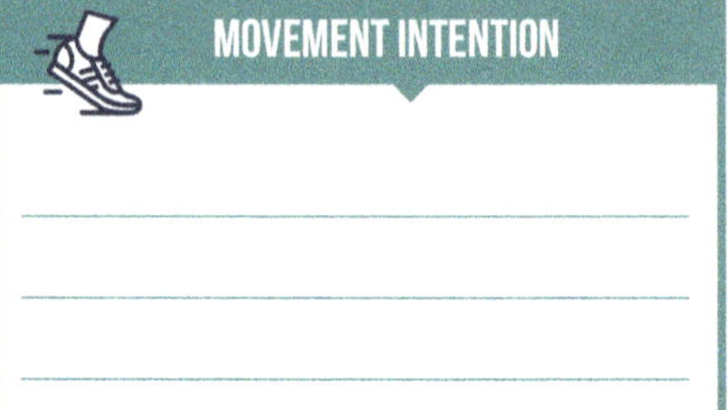

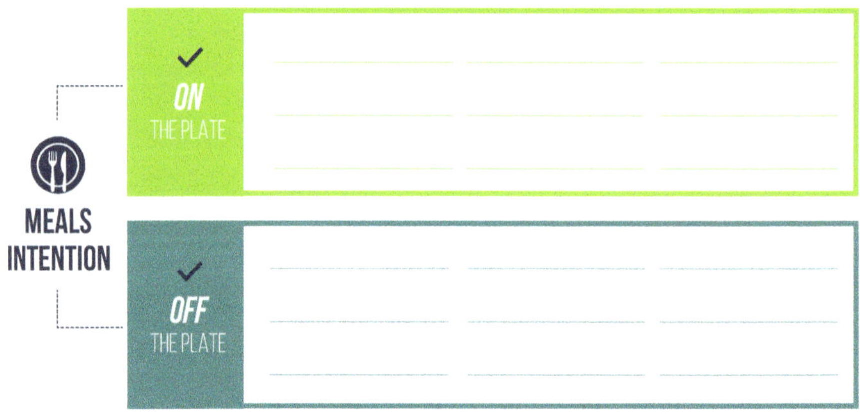

MINDFUL AFFIRMATION:

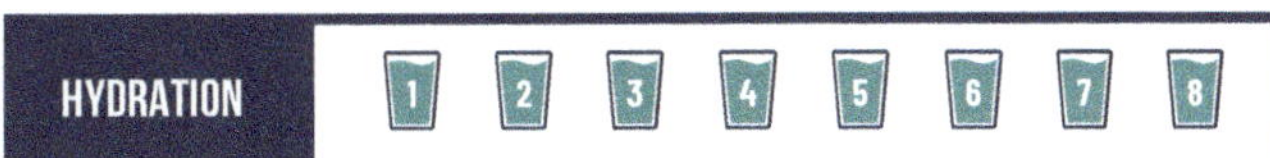

WHAT DIDN'T WORK TODAY?:

MOVEMENT:

MEALS: ON OFF

TODAY'S WINS:

1

2

3

TODAY'S TAKE AWAY:

FOOD FOR THOUGHT FOR THE DAY:

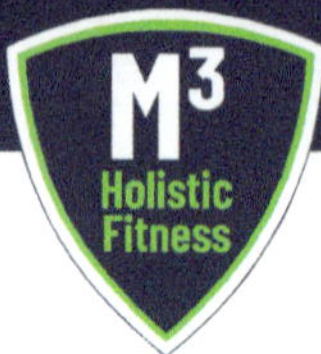

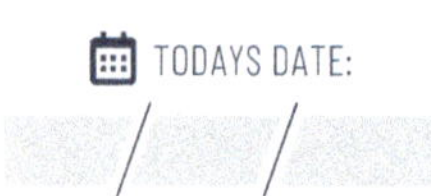

📅 **TODAYS DATE:**
____ / ____ / ____

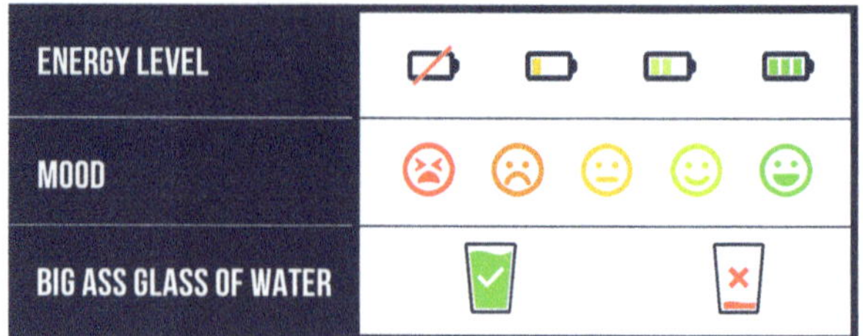

I AM GRATEFUL FOR:

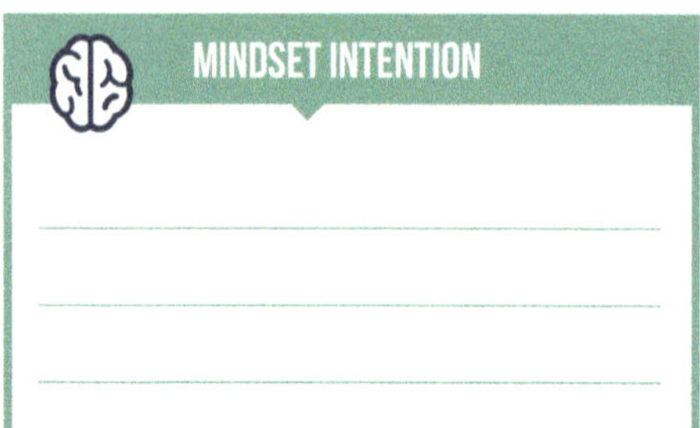

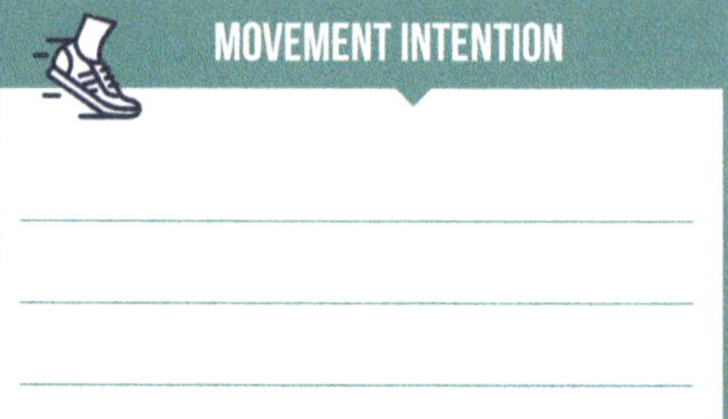

MEALS INTENTION

MINDFUL AFFIRMATION:

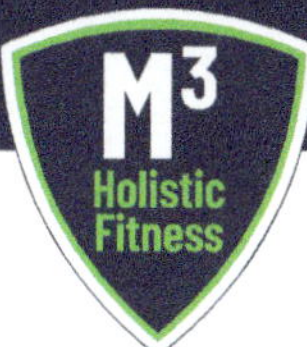

BEDTIME:

HYDRATION 1 2 3 4 5 6 7 8

WHAT DIDN'T WORK TODAY?:

MOVEMENT: ☐

MEALS: ☐ ON ☐ OFF

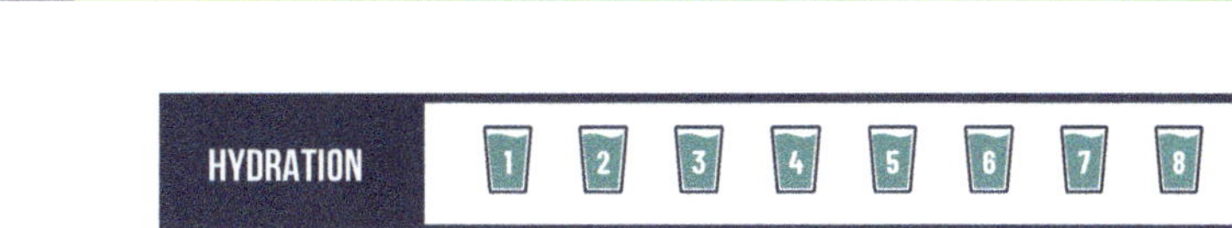

TODAY'S WINS:

1

2

3

TODAY'S TAKE AWAY:

FOOD FOR THOUGHT FOR THE DAY:

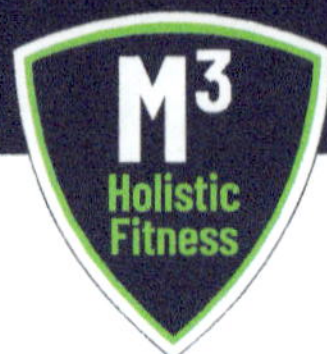

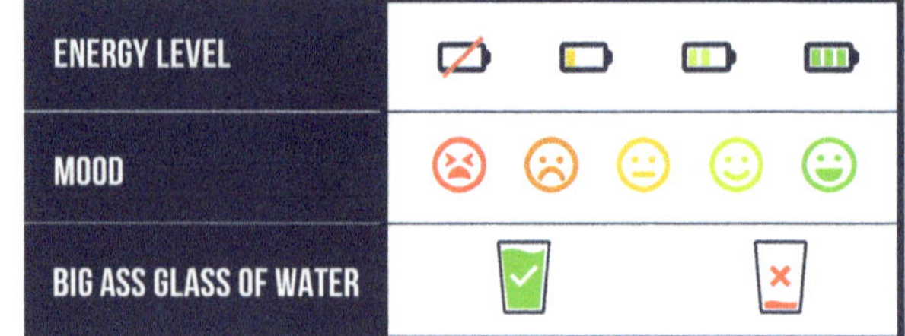

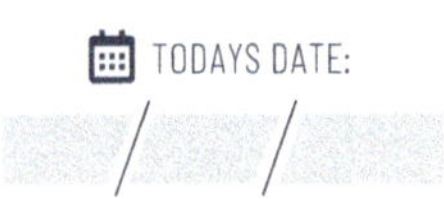

I AM GRATEFUL FOR:

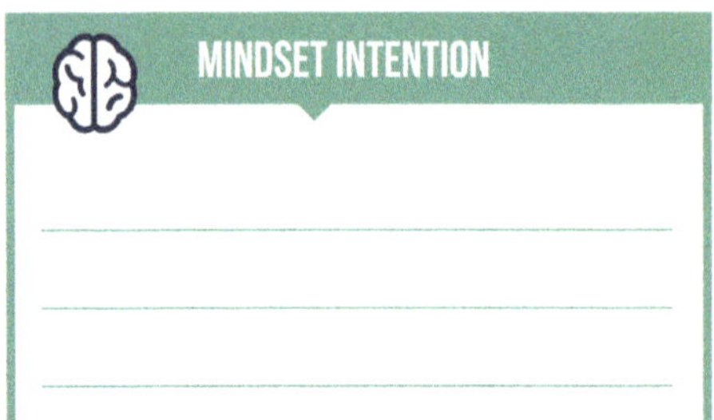

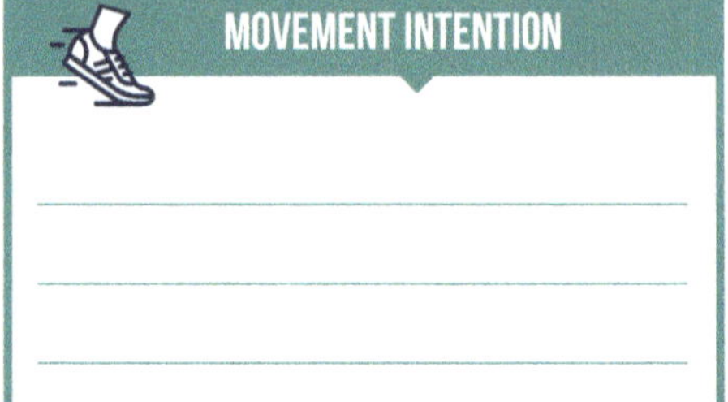

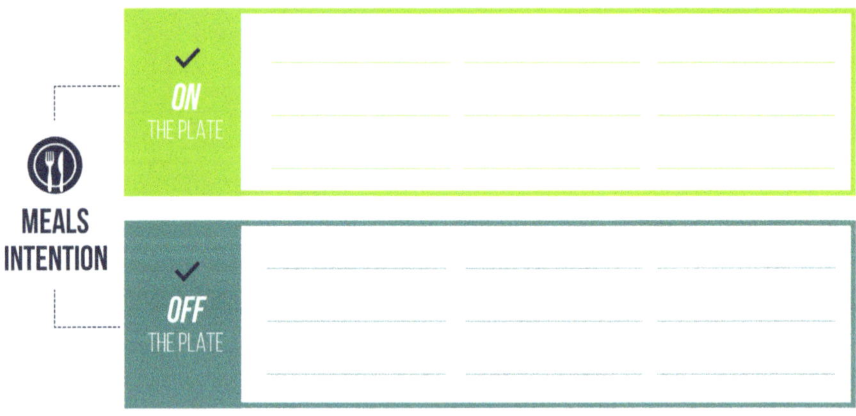

MINDFUL AFFIRMATION:

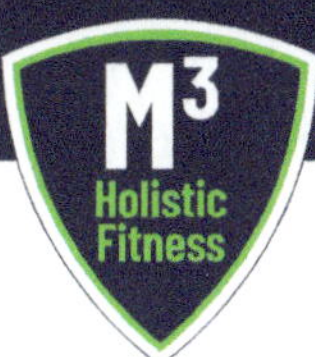

NIGHT CAP

HYDRATION 1 2 3 4 5 6 7 8

WHAT DIDN'T WORK TODAY?:

MOVEMENT:

MEALS: ON OFF

TODAY'S WINS: 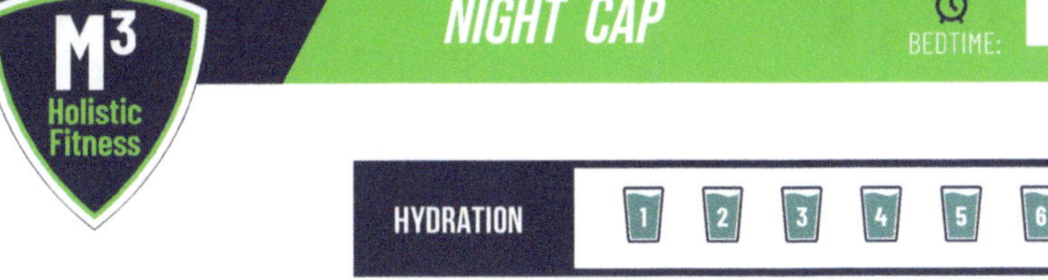

1

2

3

TODAY'S TAKE AWAY:

FOOD FOR THOUGHT FOR THE DAY:

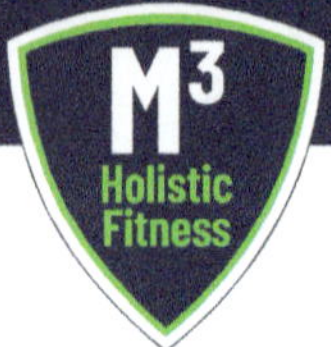

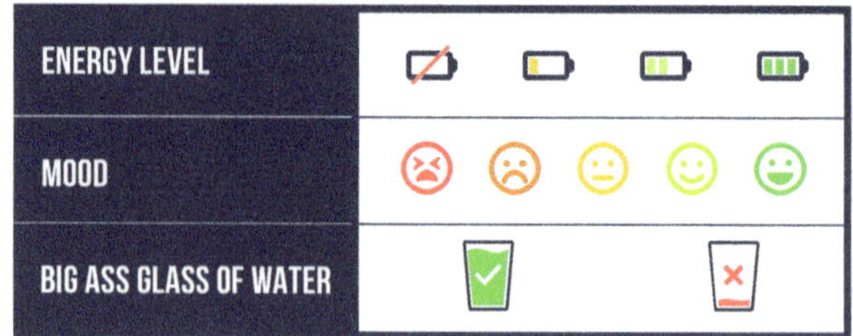

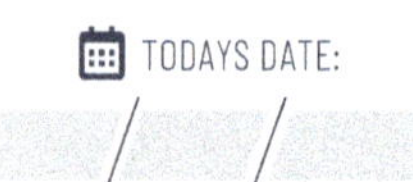

I AM GRATEFUL FOR:

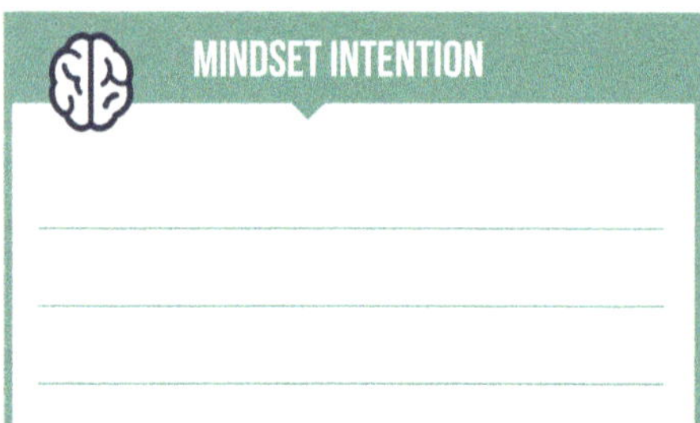

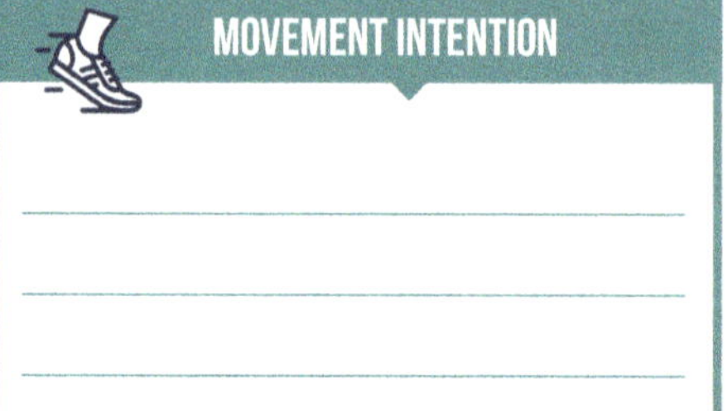

MINDFUL AFFIRMATION:

HYDRATION | 1 | 2 | 3 | 4 | 5 | 6 | 7 | 8 |

WHAT DIDN'T WORK TODAY?:

MOVEMENT: ☐

MEALS: ☐ ON ☐ OFF

TODAY'S WINS: 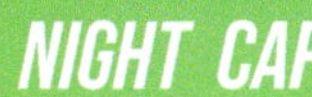

1

2

3

TODAY'S TAKE AWAY:

FOOD FOR THOUGHT FOR THE DAY:

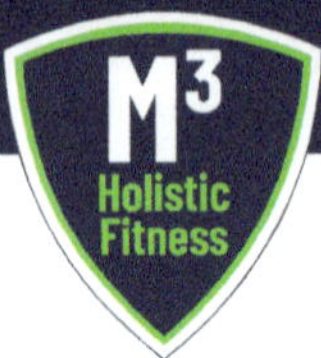

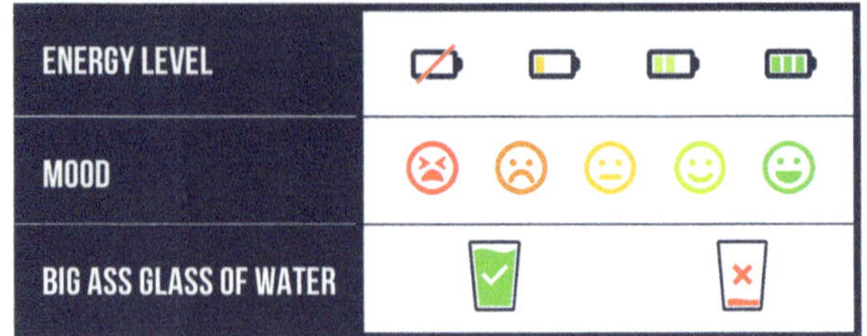

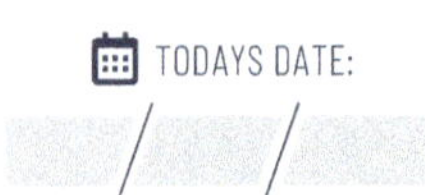

I AM GRATEFUL FOR:

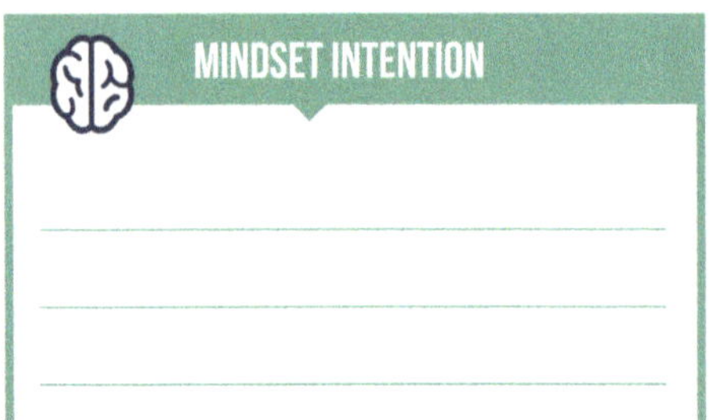

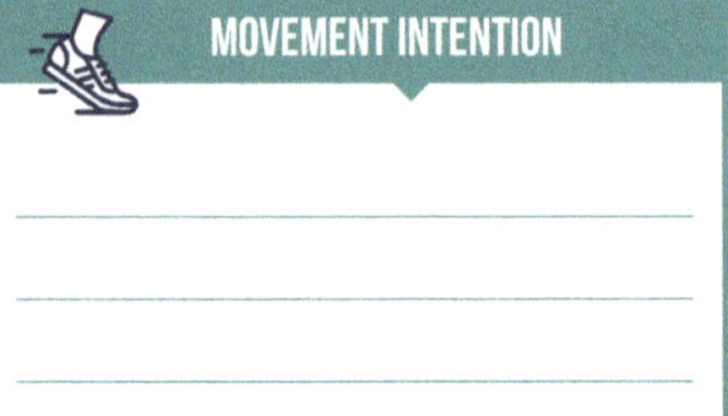

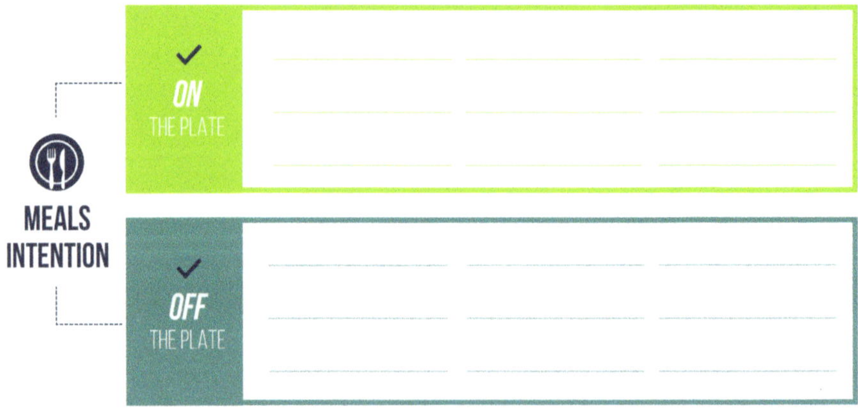

MINDFUL AFFIRMATION:

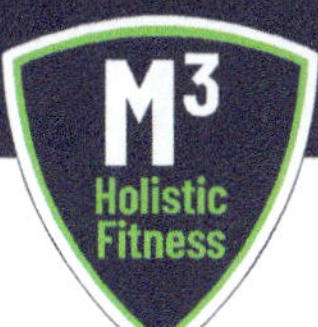

NIGHT CAP

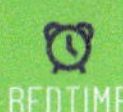

BEDTIME:

HYDRATION   1 2 3 4 5 6 7 8

WHAT DIDN'T WORK TODAY?:

MOVEMENT: ☐

MEALS: ☐ ON ☐ OFF

TODAY'S WINS: 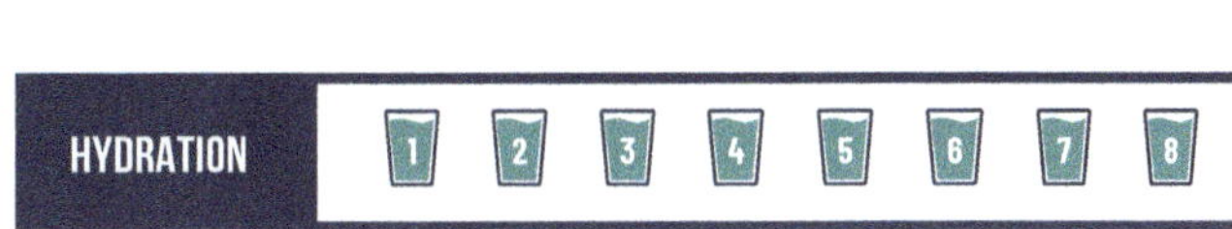

1

2

3

TODAY'S TAKE AWAY:

FOOD FOR THOUGHT FOR THE DAY:

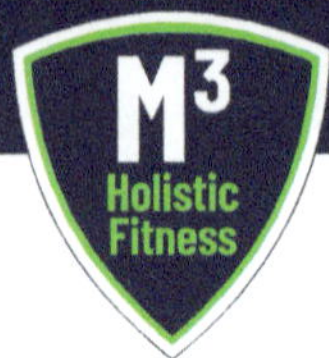

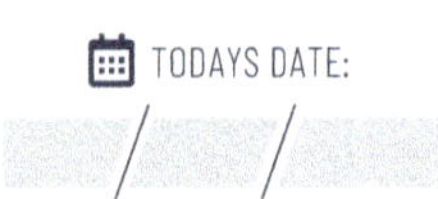

TODAYS DATE:

_____ / _____ / _____

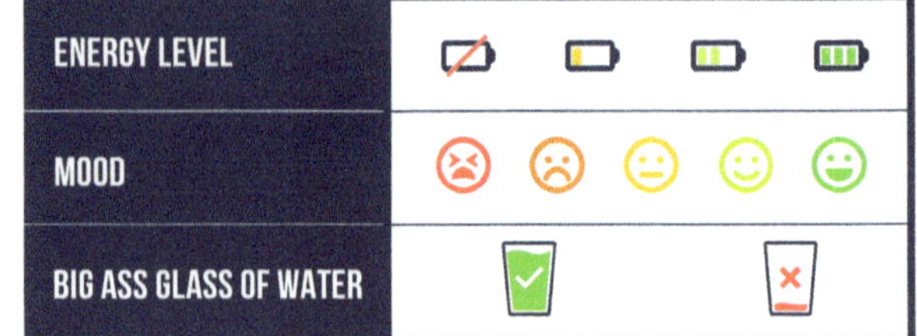

I AM GRATEFUL FOR:

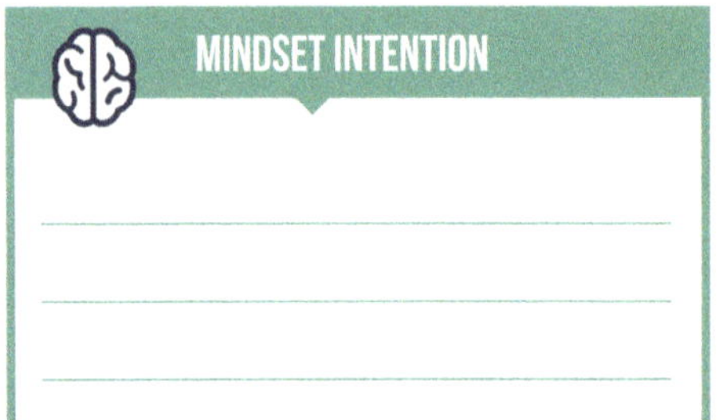

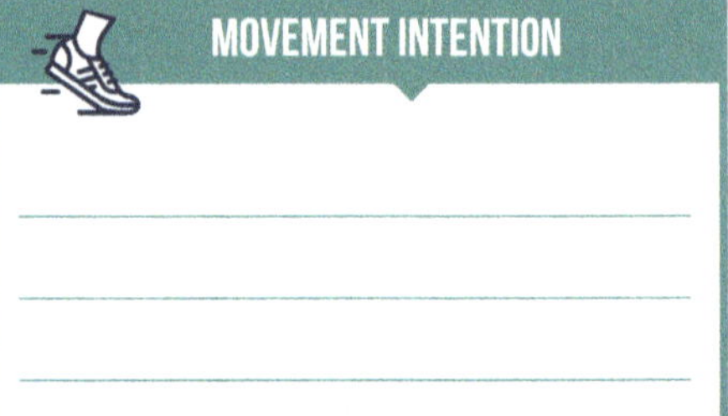

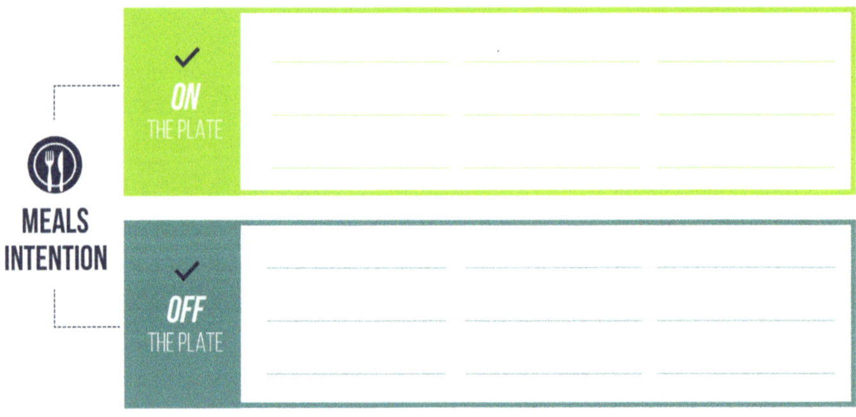

MINDFUL AFFIRMATION:

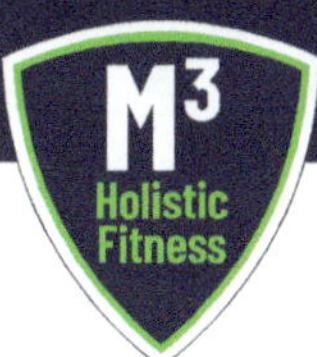

HYDRATION 1 2 3 4 5 6 7 8

WHAT DIDN'T WORK TODAY?:

MOVEMENT:

MEALS: ON OFF

TODAY'S WINS: 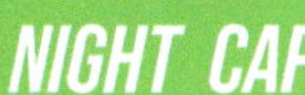

1

2

3

TODAY'S TAKE AWAY:

FOOD FOR THOUGHT FOR THE DAY:

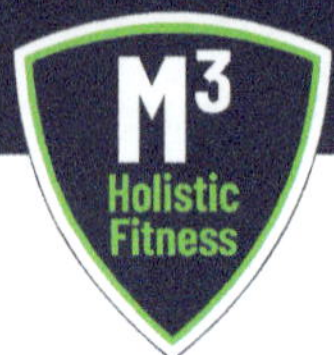

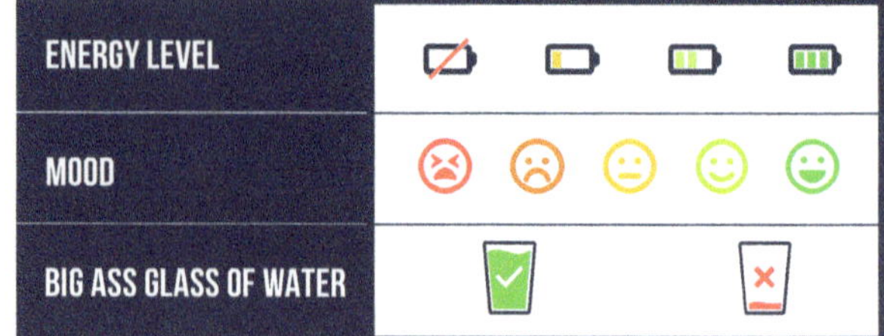

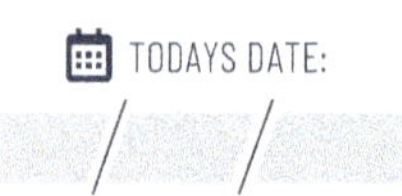

I AM GRATEFUL FOR:

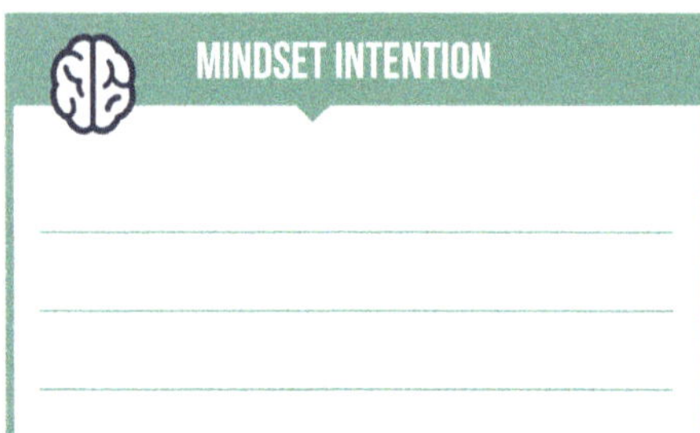

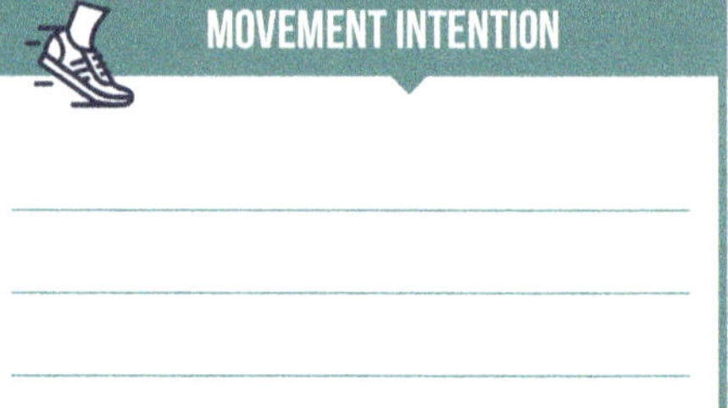

MINDFUL AFFIRMATION:

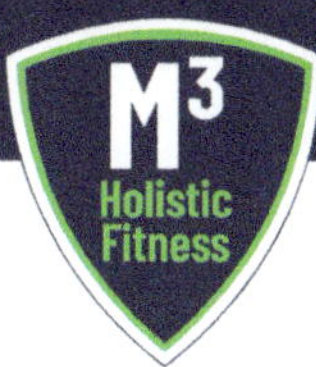

HYDRATION 1 2 3 4 5 6 7 8

WHAT DIDN'T WORK TODAY?:

MOVEMENT: ☐

MEALS: ☐ ON ☐ OFF

TODAY'S WINS:

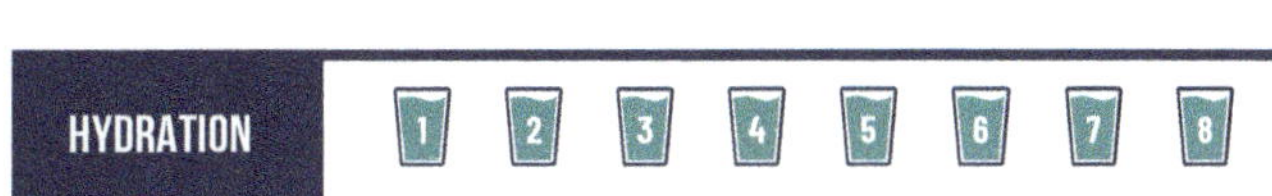

1

2

3

TODAY'S TAKE AWAY:

FOOD FOR THOUGHT FOR THE DAY:

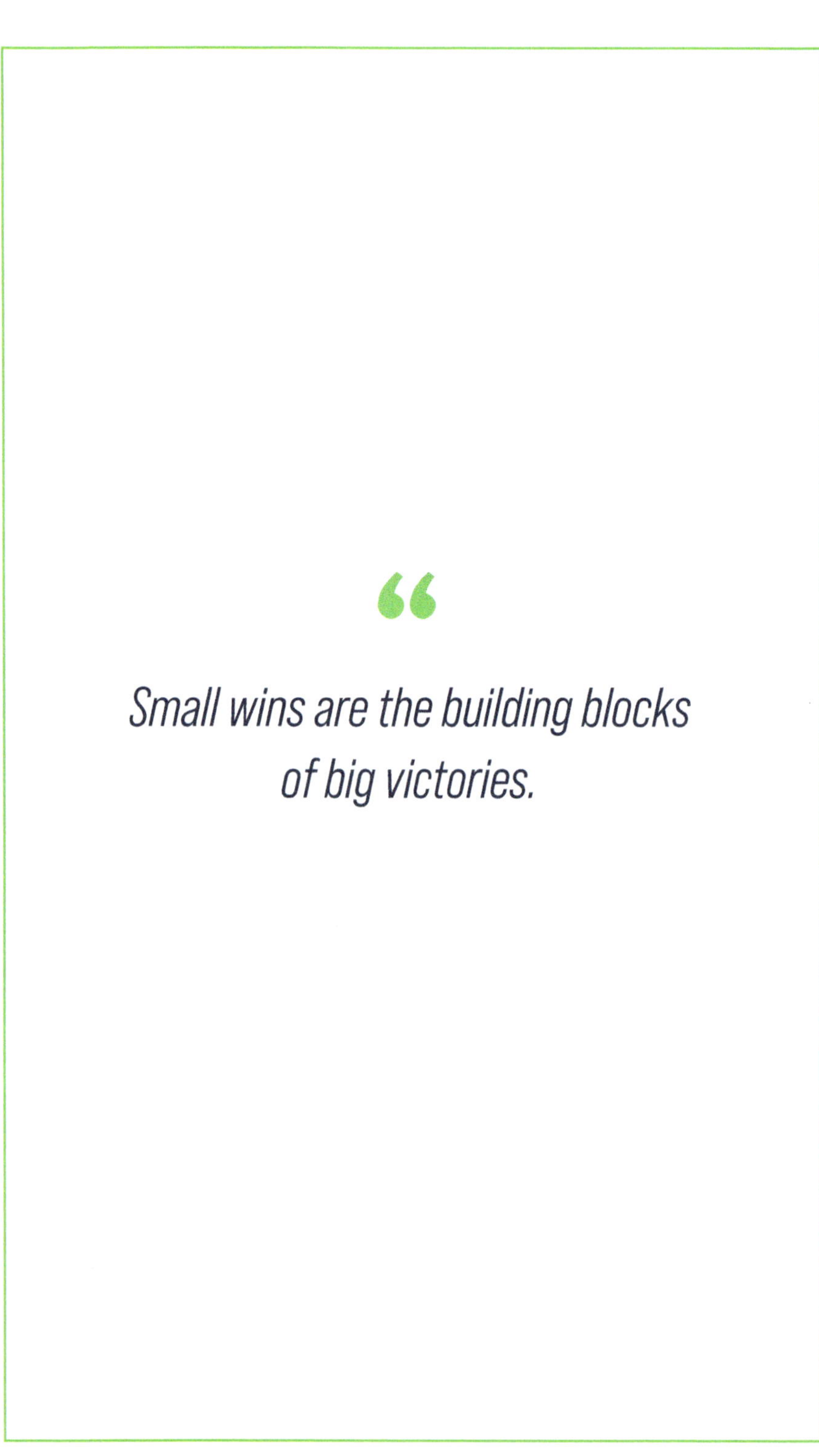

Small wins are the building blocks
of big victories.

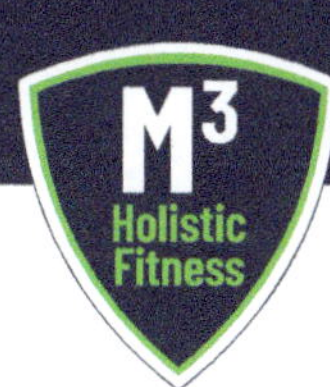

THIS WEEKS WINS:

THIS WEEKS TAKEAWAYS:

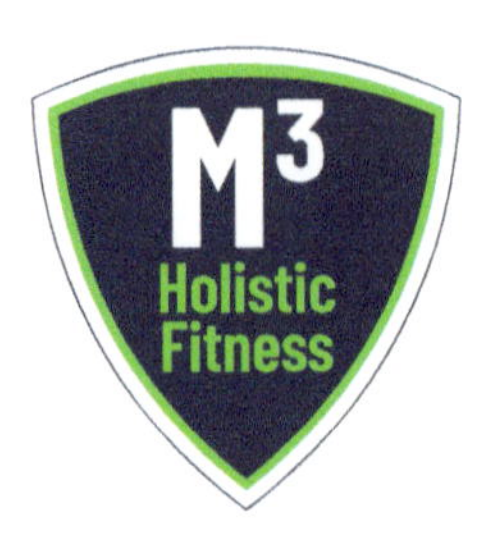

WEEK 7

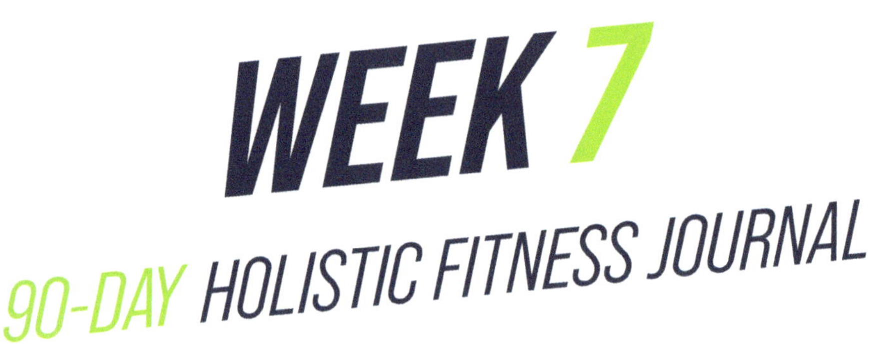

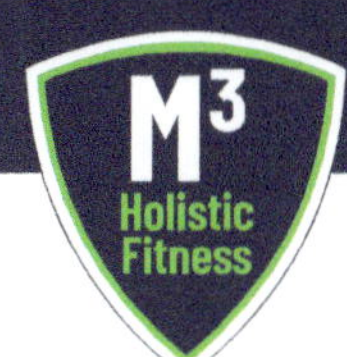

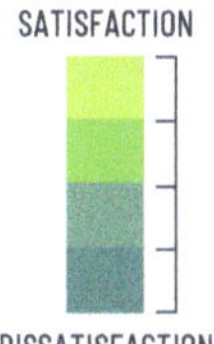

SATISFACTION

DISSATISFACTION

EXAMPLE

WHAT DOES YOUR LIFE LOOK LIKE?

1. Place a dot in each category to indicate your level of satisfaction within each area. A dot at the **center of the circle to indicate dissatisfaction,** or towards the **outer edge to indicate satisfaction.** Most people fall somewhere in between. (see example)

2. Connect the dots to see your **M₃ Circle of Life.**

3. Identify imbalances. Determine where to spend more time and energy to create balance. **This will help you create a better balance for your best Badass Life.**

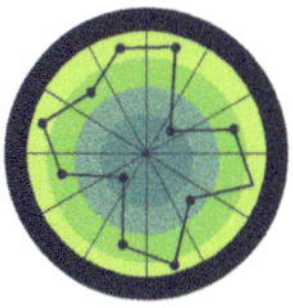

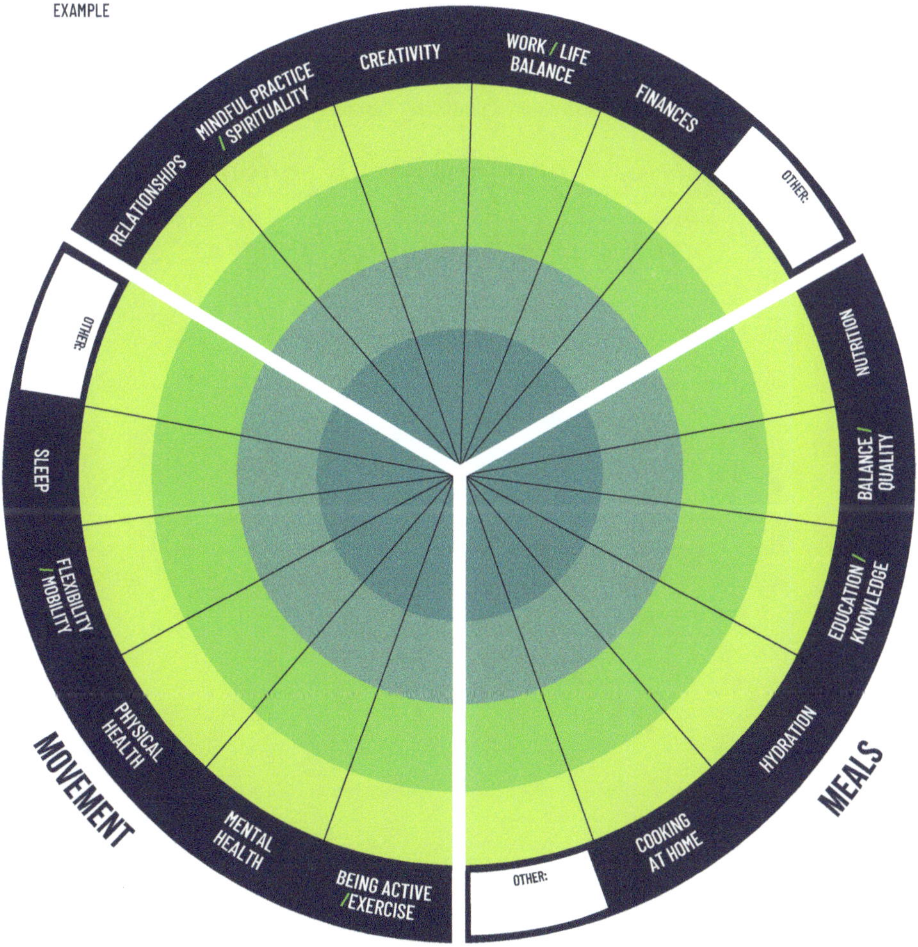

"

*The decisions you make today
are the results you will see
tomorrow.*

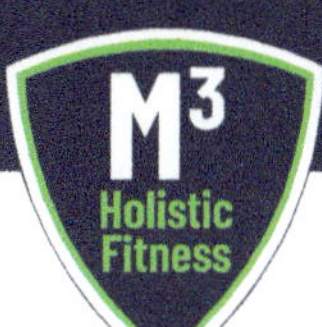

MAKE IT HAPPEN THIS WEEK

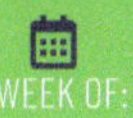 WEEK OF: ___ / ___ / ___

	MINDSET	MOVEMENT	MEALS	
			✓ ON THE PLATE	✓ OFF THE PLATE
MON				
TUES				
WEDS				
THURS				
FRI				
SAT				
SUN				

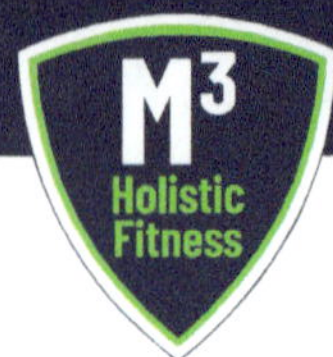

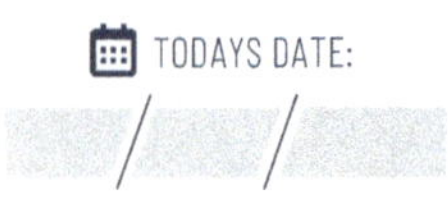

⏰ WAKE UP: _______   SLEEP: ___ Hrs

📅 TODAYS DATE: ____ / ____ / ____

ENERGY LEVEL				
MOOD				
BIG ASS GLASS OF WATER	✅		✖	

I AM GRATEFUL FOR:

____

____

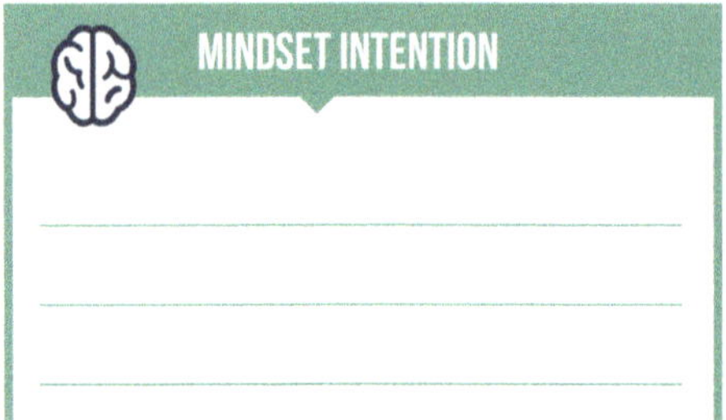

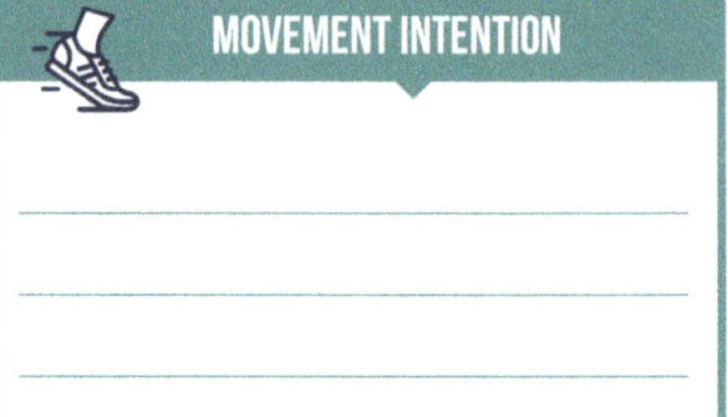

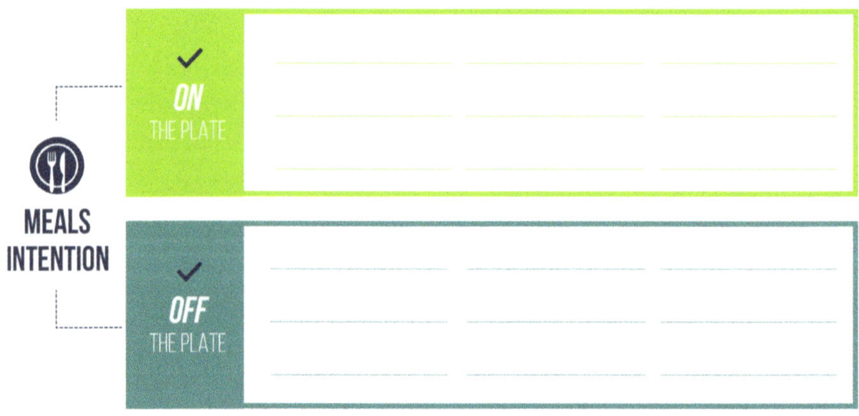

MINDFUL AFFIRMATION:

____

____

HYDRATION   1 2 3 4 5 6 7 8

WHAT DIDN'T WORK TODAY?:

MOVEMENT: ☐

MEALS: ☐ ON ☐ OFF

TODAY'S WINS:

1

2

3

TODAY'S TAKE AWAY:

FOOD FOR THOUGHT FOR THE DAY:

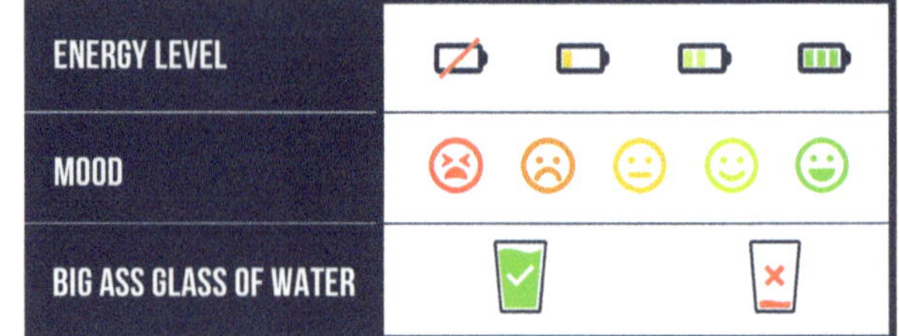

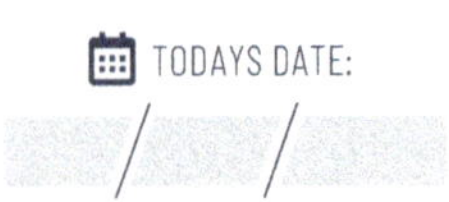

ENERGY LEVEL				
MOOD				
BIG ASS GLASS OF WATER				

I AM GRATEFUL FOR:

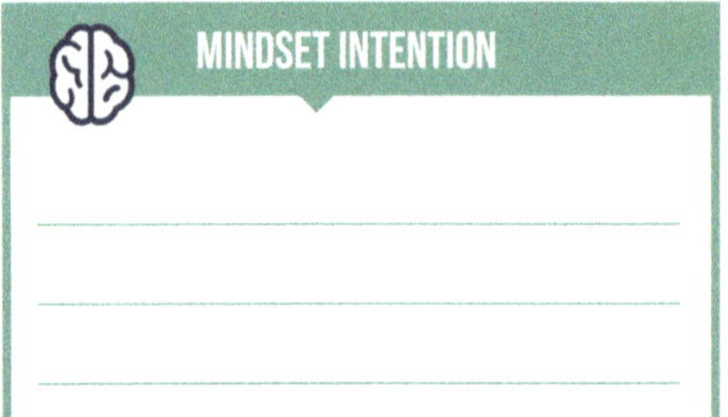

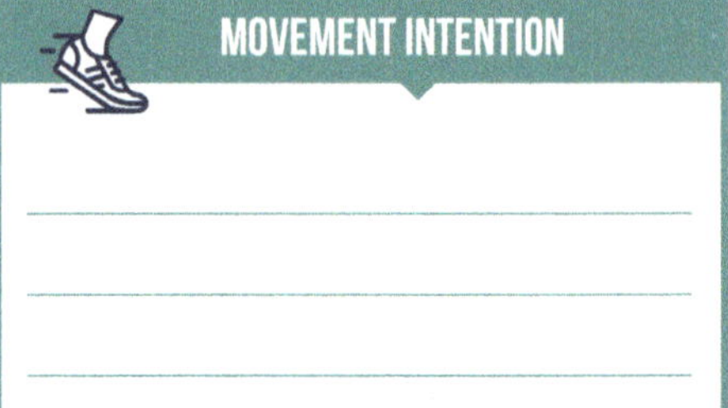

MINDFUL AFFIRMATION:

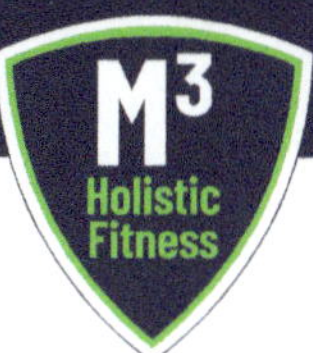

BEDTIME:

HYDRATION 1 2 3 4 5 6 7 8

WHAT DIDN'T WORK TODAY?:

MOVEMENT: ☐

MEALS: ☐ ON ☐ OFF

TODAY'S WINS: 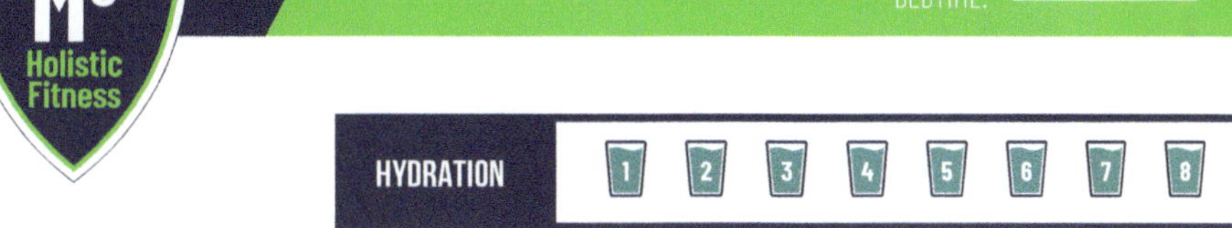

1

2

3

TODAY'S TAKE AWAY:

FOOD FOR THOUGHT FOR THE DAY:

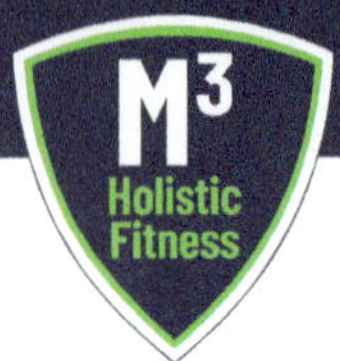

RISE AND ALIGN

WAKE UP: ___________   SLEEP: _____ Hrs

ENERGY LEVEL				
MOOD				
BIG ASS GLASS OF WATER				

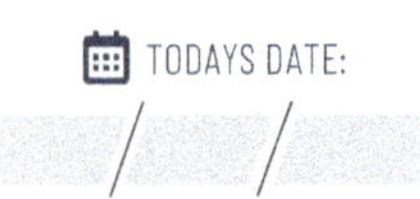 TODAYS DATE: ______ / ______ / ______

I AM GRATEFUL FOR:

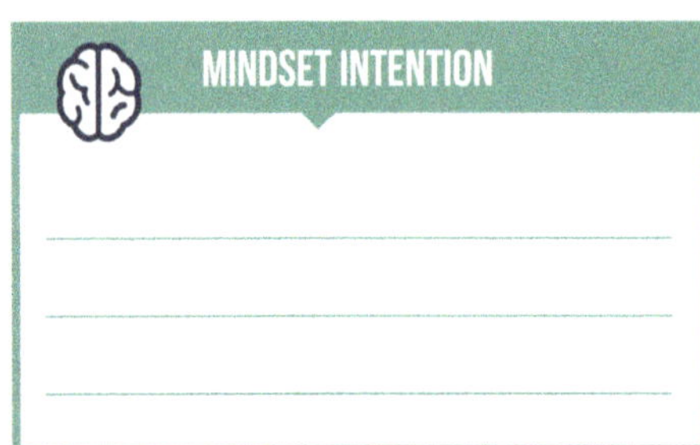

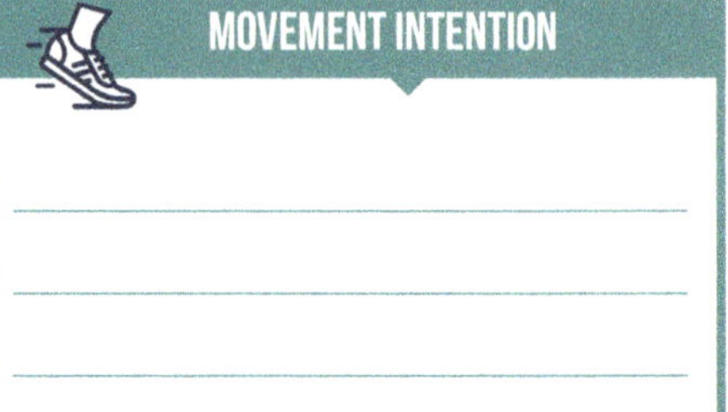

MINDFUL AFFIRMATION:

NIGHT CAP

BEDTIME:

HYDRATION 1 2 3 4 5 6 7 8

WHAT DIDN'T WORK TODAY?:

MOVEMENT:

MEALS: ON OFF

TODAY'S WINS:

1

2

3

TODAY'S TAKE AWAY:

FOOD FOR THOUGHT FOR THE DAY:

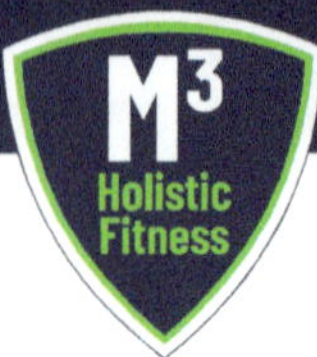

TODAYS DATE: ___ / ___ / ___

ENERGY LEVEL				
MOOD				
BIG ASS GLASS OF WATER				

I AM GRATEFUL FOR:

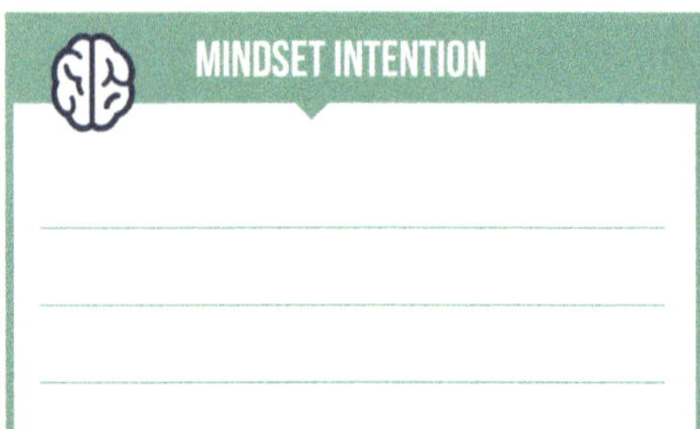

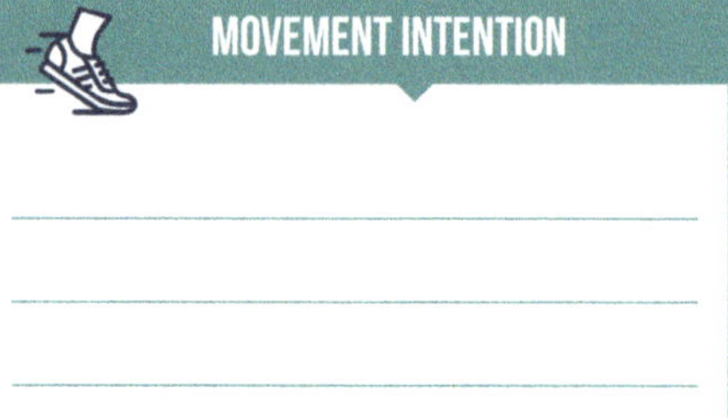

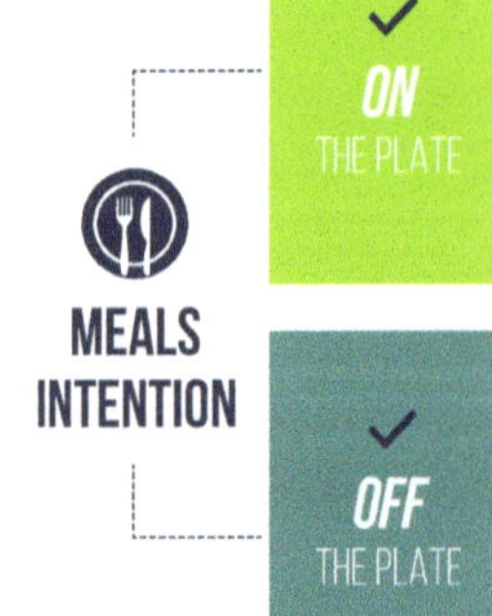

ON
THE PLATE

OFF
THE PLATE

MINDFUL AFFIRMATION:

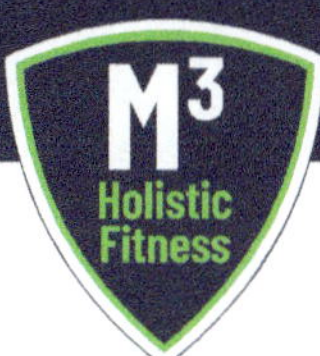

NIGHT CAP

BEDTIME:

HYDRATION 1 2 3 4 5 6 7 8

WHAT DIDN'T WORK TODAY?:

MOVEMENT: ☐

MEALS: ☐ ON ☐ OFF

TODAY'S WINS: 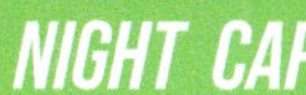

1

2

3

TODAY'S TAKE AWAY:

FOOD FOR THOUGHT FOR THE DAY:

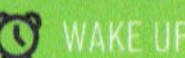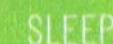

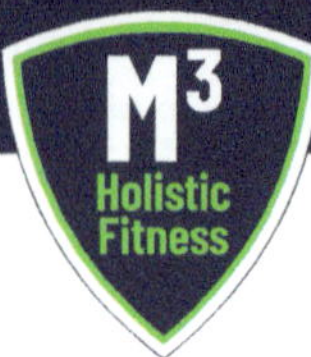

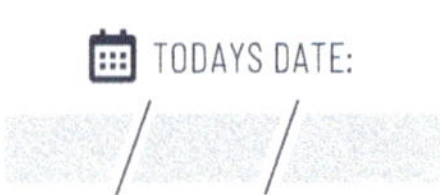

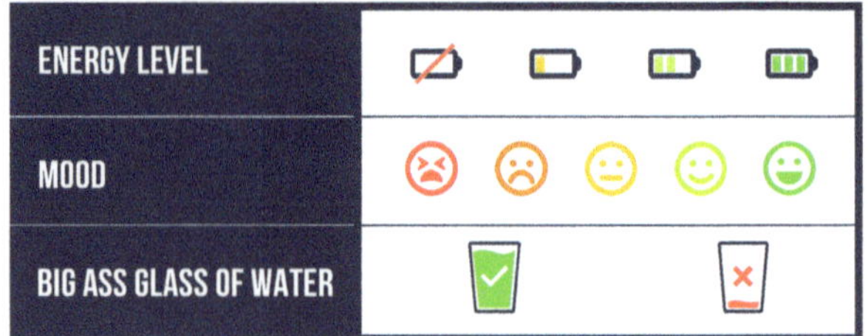

I AM GRATEFUL FOR:

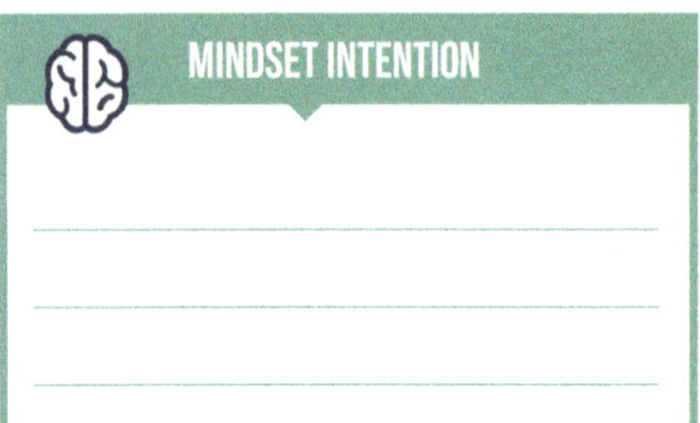

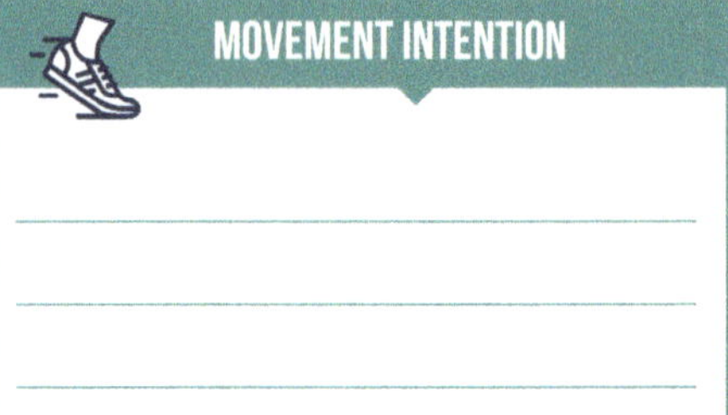

MINDFUL AFFIRMATION:

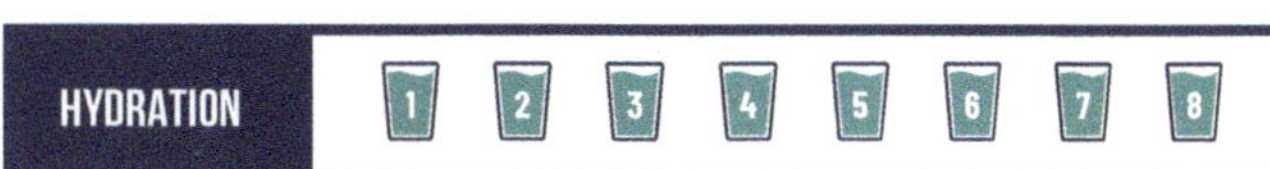

HYDRATION 1 2 3 4 5 6 7 8

WHAT DIDN'T WORK TODAY?:

MOVEMENT: ☐

MEALS: ☐ ON ☐ OFF

TODAY'S WINS:

1

2

3

TODAY'S TAKE AWAY:

FOOD FOR THOUGHT FOR THE DAY:

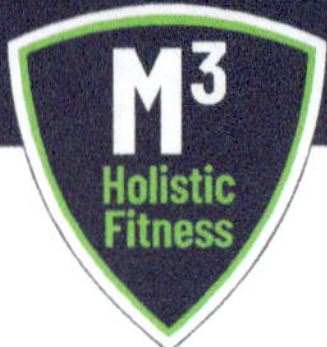

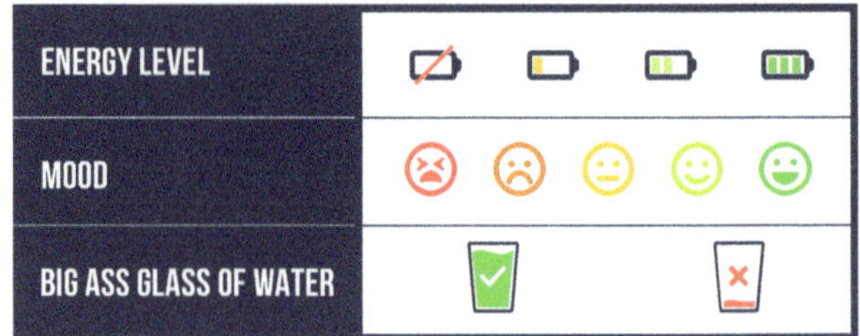

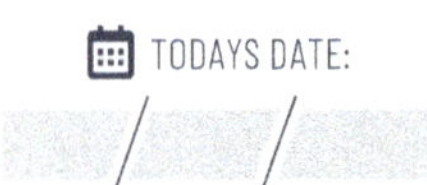

ENERGY LEVEL				
MOOD				
BIG ASS GLASS OF WATER				

I AM GRATEFUL FOR:

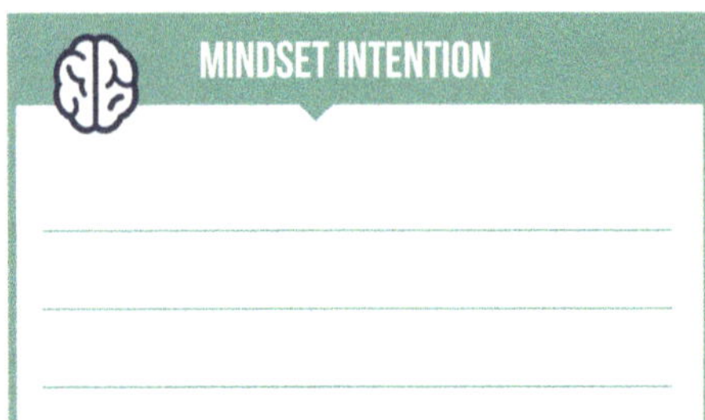

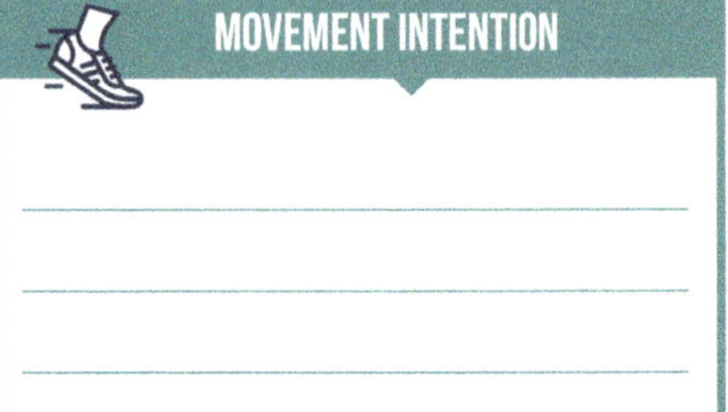

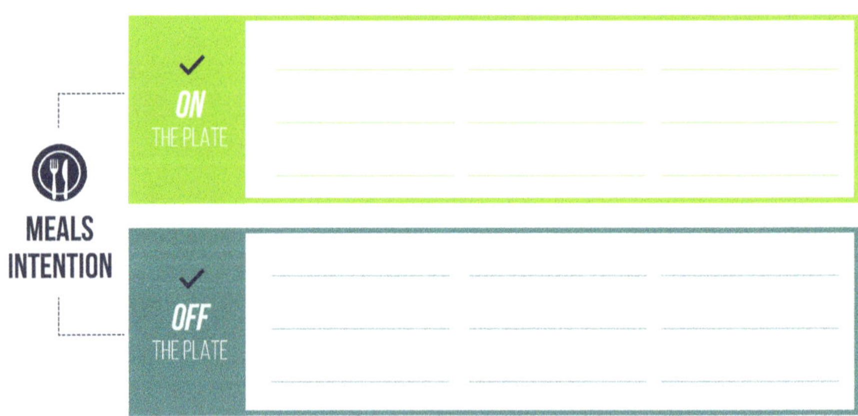

MINDFUL AFFIRMATION:

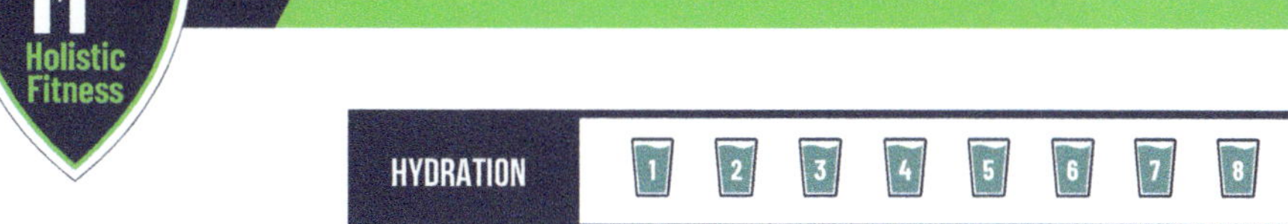

HYDRATION | 1 | 2 | 3 | 4 | 5 | 6 | 7 | 8 |

WHAT DIDN'T WORK TODAY?:

MOVEMENT: ☐

MEALS: ☐ ON ☐ OFF

TODAY'S WINS:

| 1 | 2 | 3 |

TODAY'S TAKE AWAY:

FOOD FOR THOUGHT FOR THE DAY:

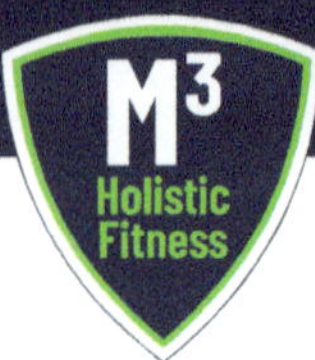

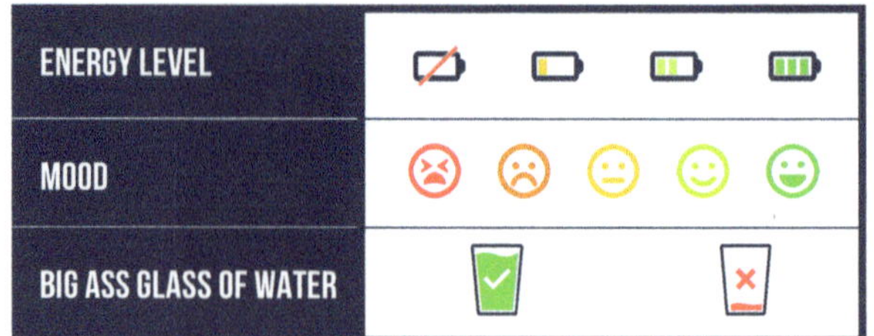

ENERGY LEVEL				
MOOD				
BIG ASS GLASS OF WATER				

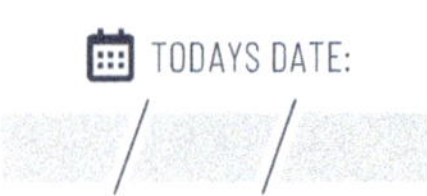

TODAYS DATE: ___ / ___ / ___

I AM GRATEFUL FOR:

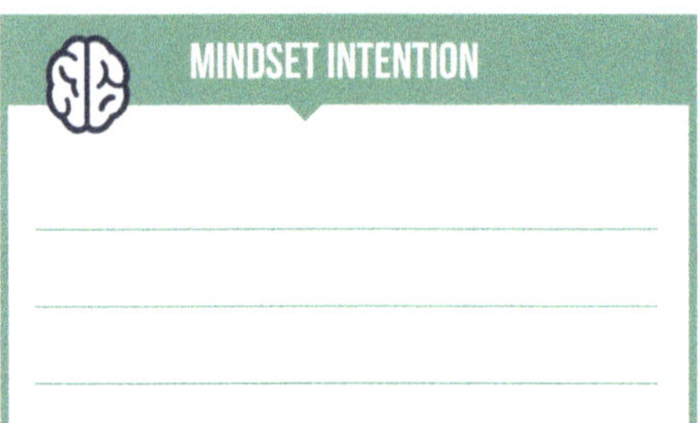

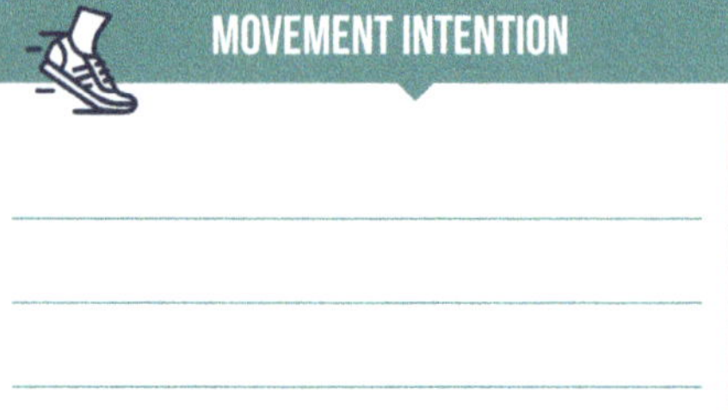

MINDFUL AFFIRMATION:

HYDRATION 1 2 3 4 5 6 7 8

WHAT DIDN'T WORK TODAY?:

MOVEMENT: ☐

MEALS: ☐ ON ☐ OFF

TODAY'S WINS:

1

2

3

TODAY'S TAKE AWAY:

FOOD FOR THOUGHT FOR THE DAY:

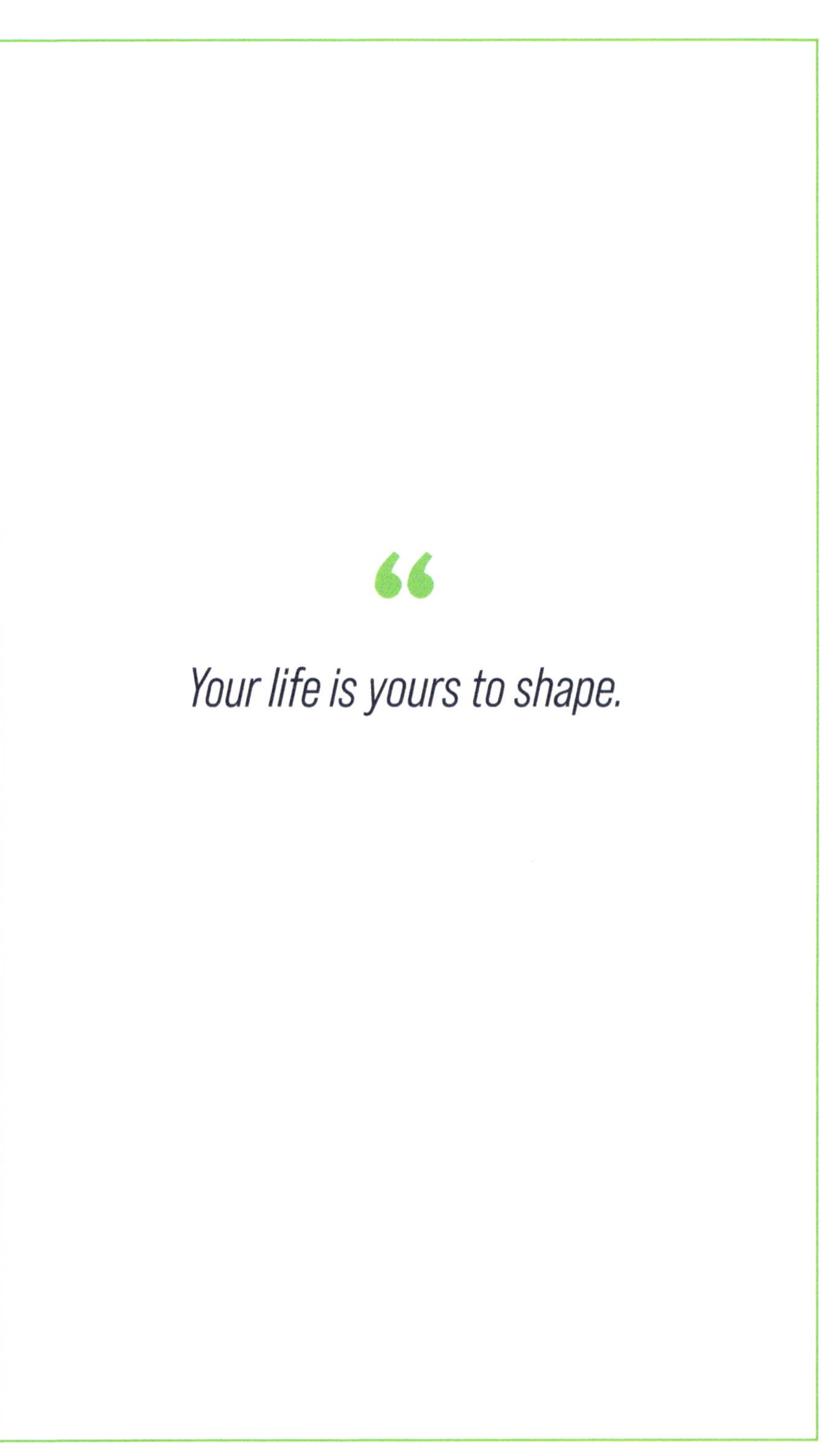

"
Your life is yours to shape.

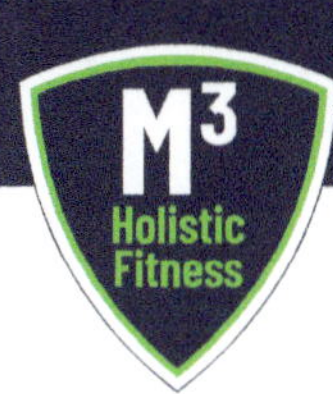

THIS WEEKS WINS:

THIS WEEKS TAKEAWAYS:

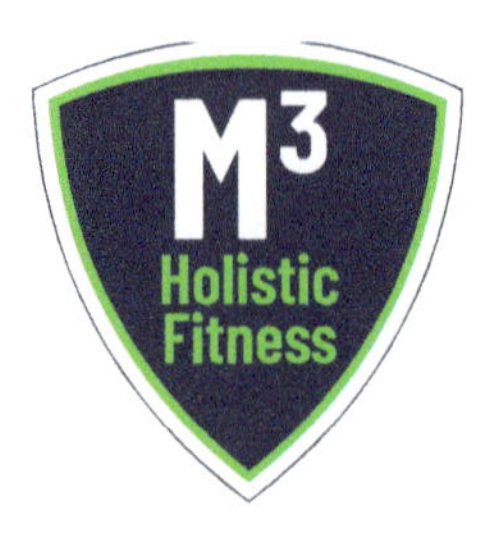

WEEK 8

90-DAY HOLISTIC FITNESS JOURNAL

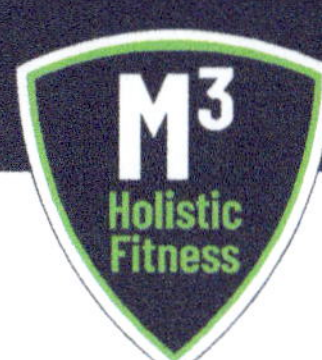

WHAT DOES *YOUR* LIFE LOOK LIKE?

SATISFACTION

DISSATISFACTION

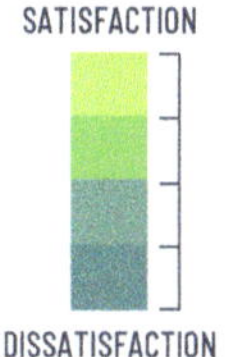

EXAMPLE

1. Place a dot in each category to indicate your level of satisfaction within each area. A dot at the **center of the circle to indicate dissatisfaction**, or towards the **outer edge to indicate satisfaction**. Most people fall somewhere in between. (see example)

2. Connect the dots to see your **M₃ Circle of Life**.

3. Identify imbalances. Determine where to spend more time and energy to create balance. **This will help you create a better balance for your best Badass Life.**

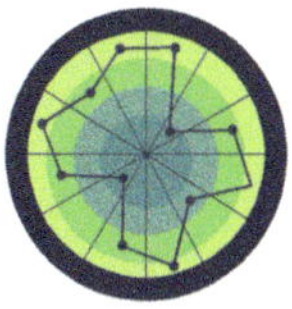

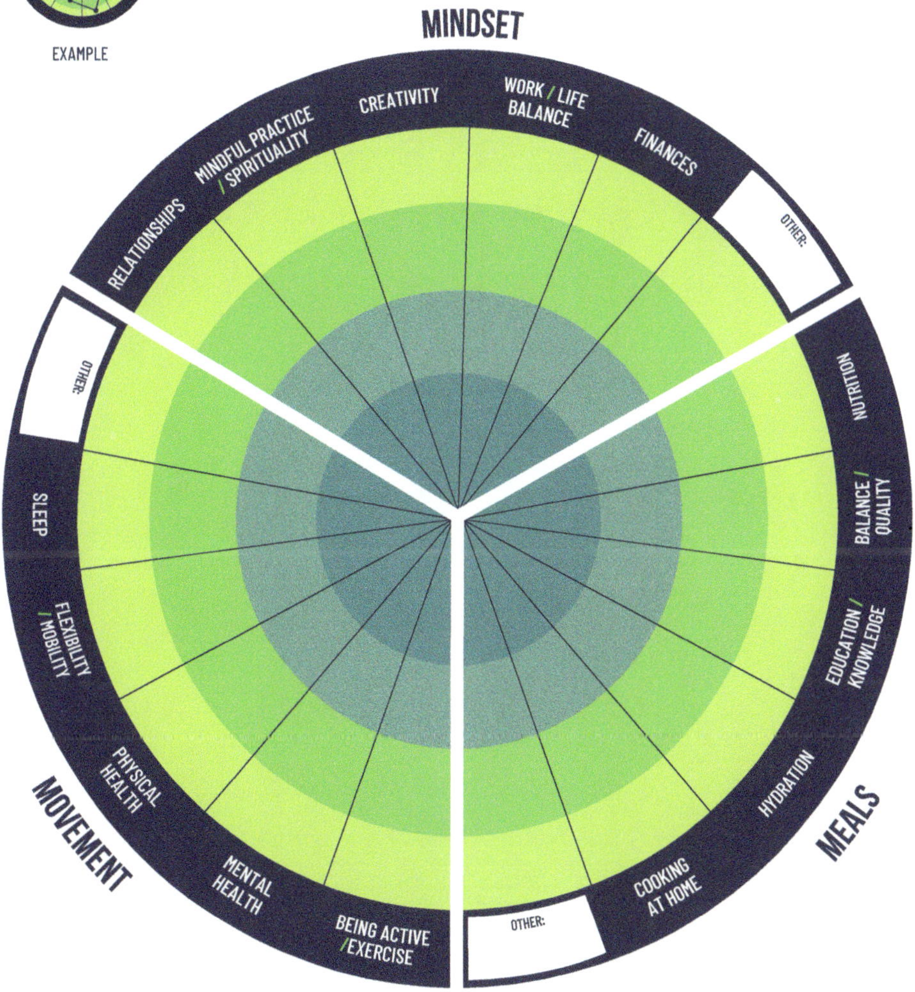

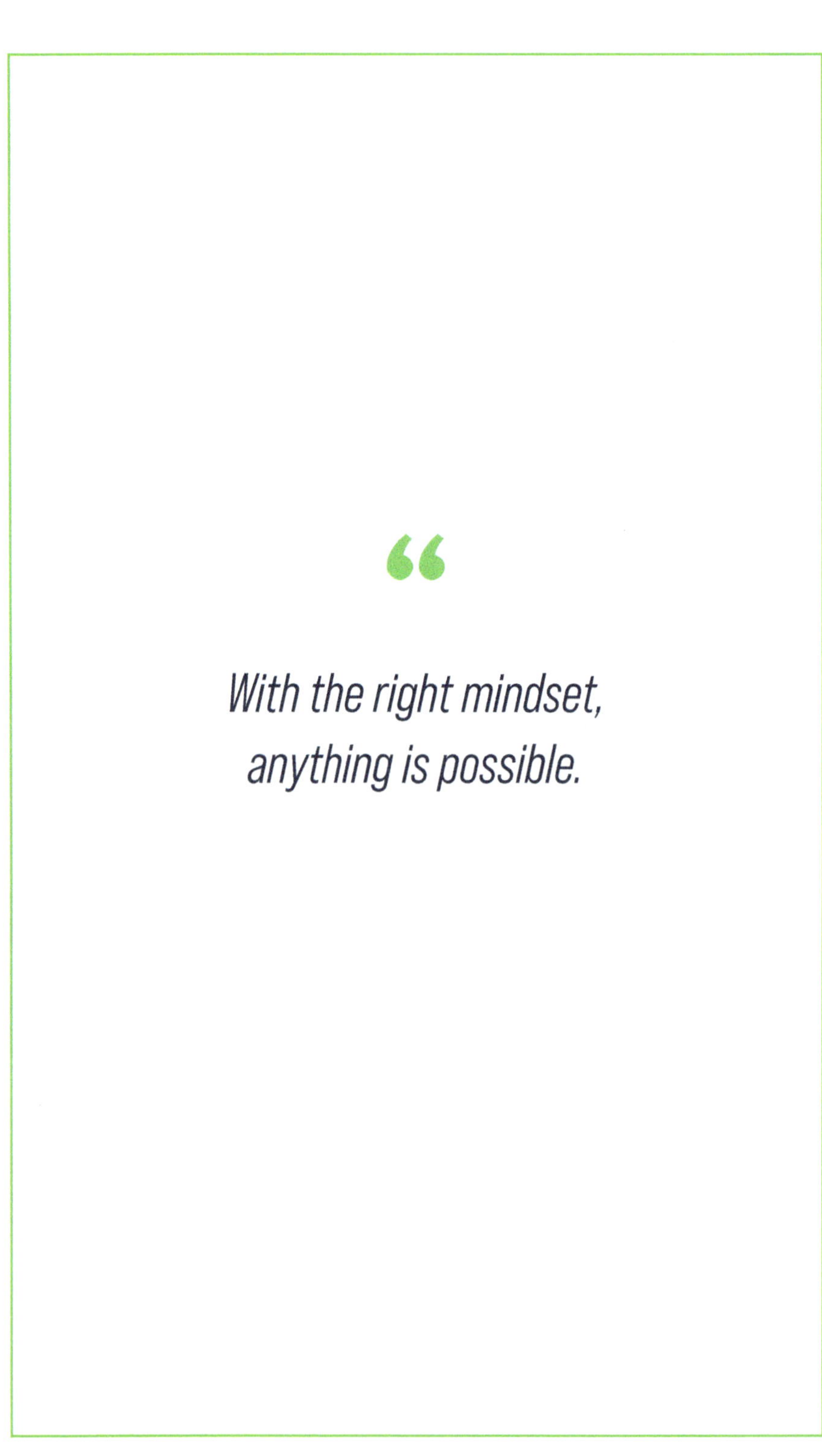

With the right mindset,
anything is possible.

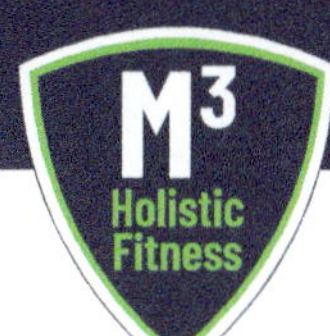

WEEK OF: ___ / ___ / ___

	MINDSET	MOVEMENT	MEALS — ON THE PLATE	MEALS — OFF THE PLATE
MON				
TUES				
WEDS				
THURS				
FRI				
SAT				
SUN				

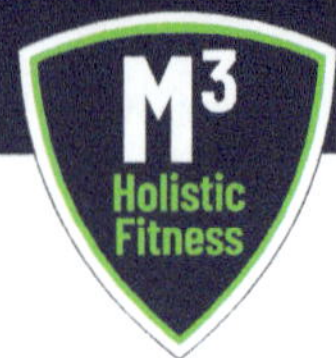

WAKE UP:

SLEEP: Hrs

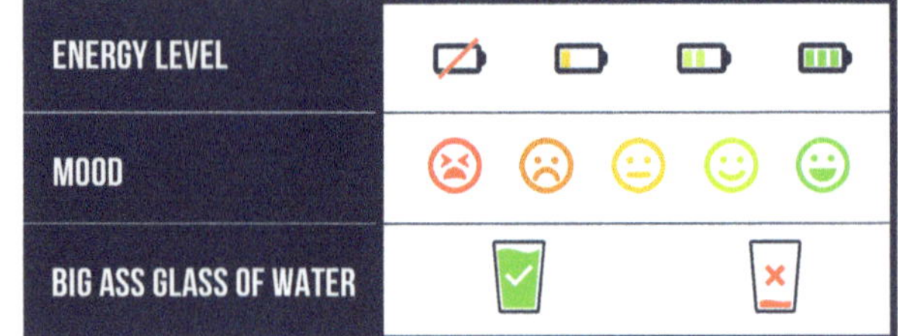

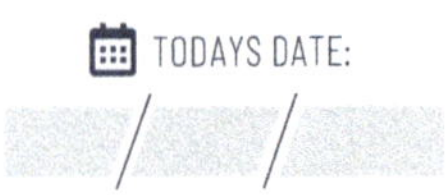

I AM GRATEFUL FOR:

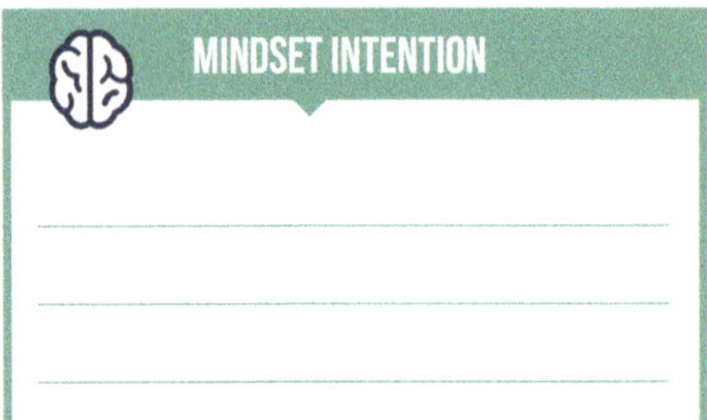

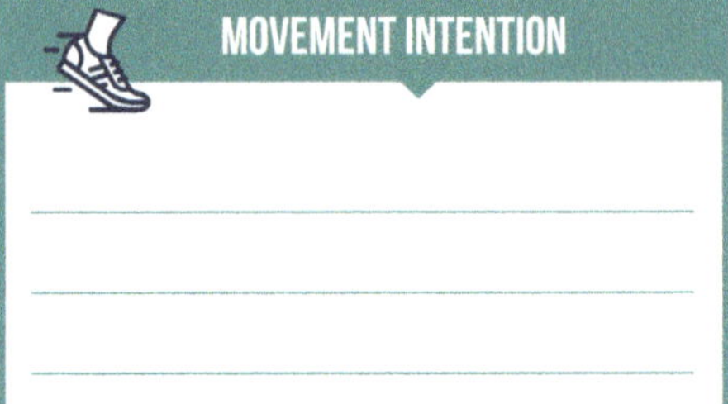

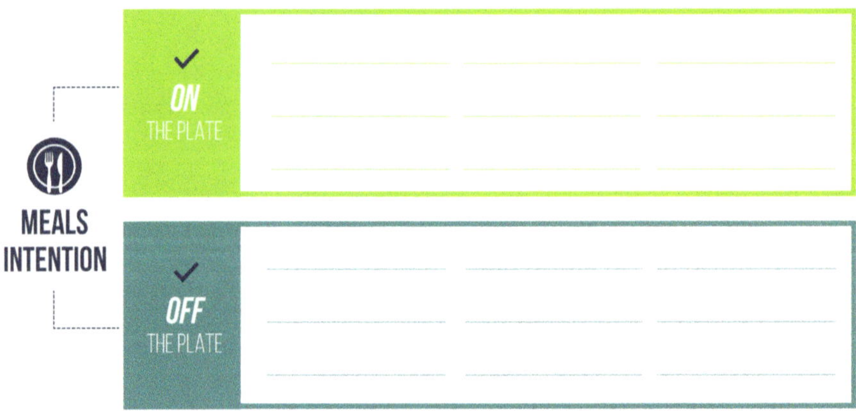

MINDFUL AFFIRMATION:

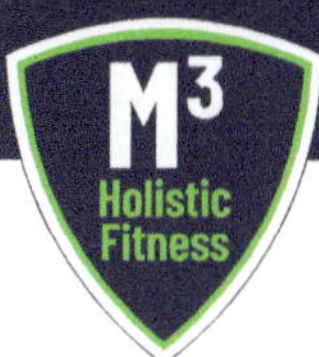

HYDRATION 1 2 3 4 5 6 7 8

WHAT DIDN'T WORK TODAY?:

MOVEMENT: ☐

MEALS: ☐ ON ☐ OFF

TODAY'S WINS: 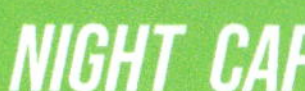

1

2

3

TODAY'S TAKE AWAY:

FOOD FOR THOUGHT FOR THE DAY:

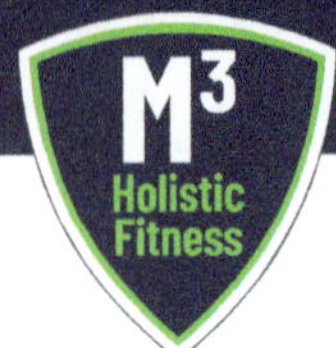

M³
Holistic Fitness

TODAYS DATE:

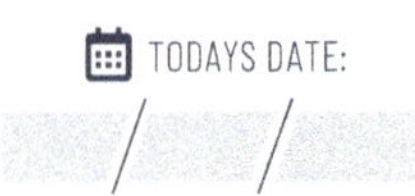

ENERGY LEVEL				
MOOD				
BIG ASS GLASS OF WATER				

I AM GRATEFUL FOR:

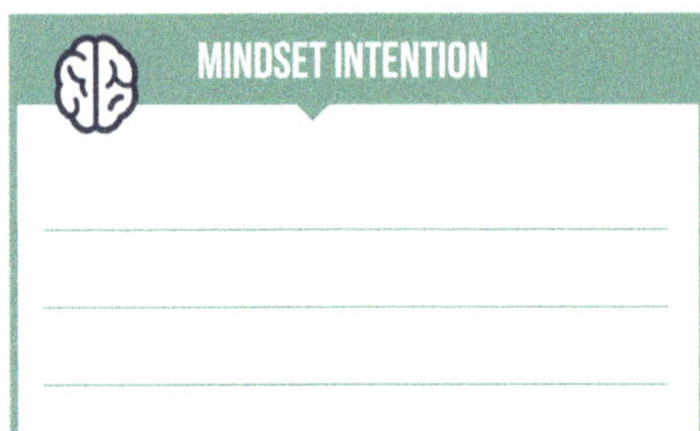

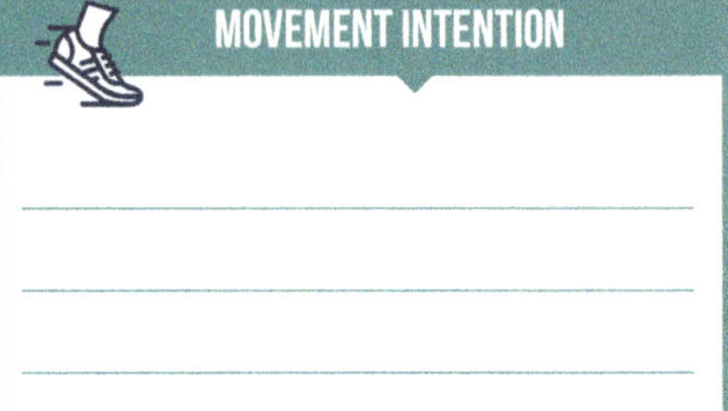

MINDFUL AFFIRMATION:

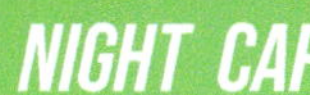
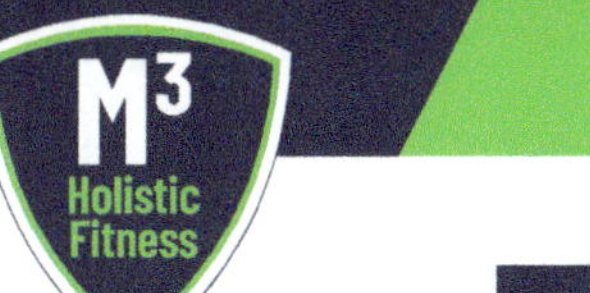

NIGHT CAP

BEDTIME:

HYDRATION 1 2 3 4 5 6 7 8

WHAT DIDN'T WORK TODAY?:

MOVEMENT: ☐

MEALS: ☐ ON ☐ OFF

TODAY'S WINS:

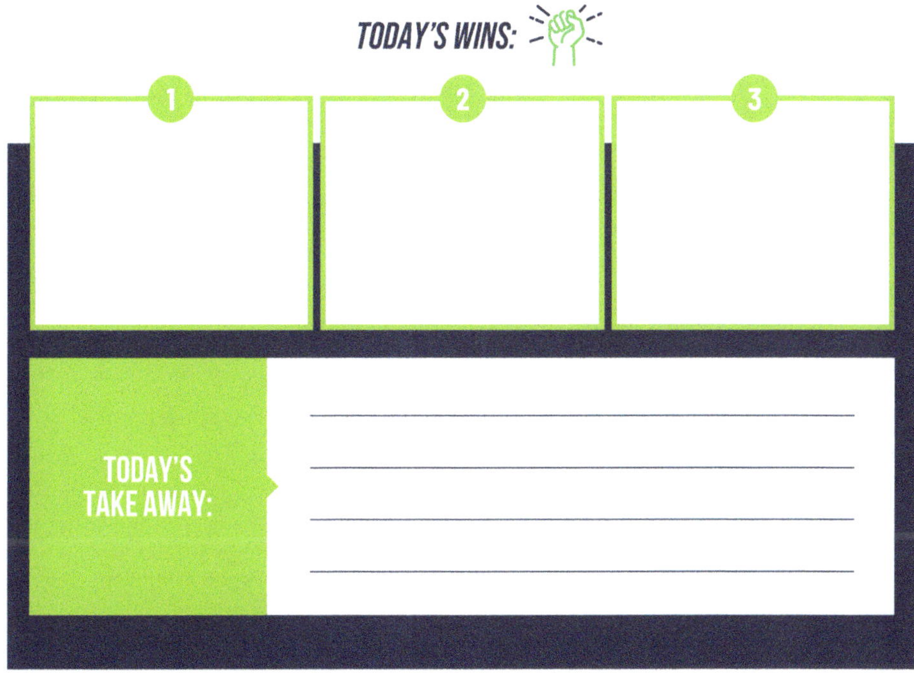

1

2

3

TODAY'S TAKE AWAY:

FOOD FOR THOUGHT FOR THE DAY:

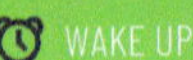

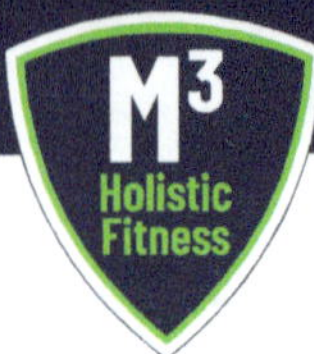

TODAYS DATE:

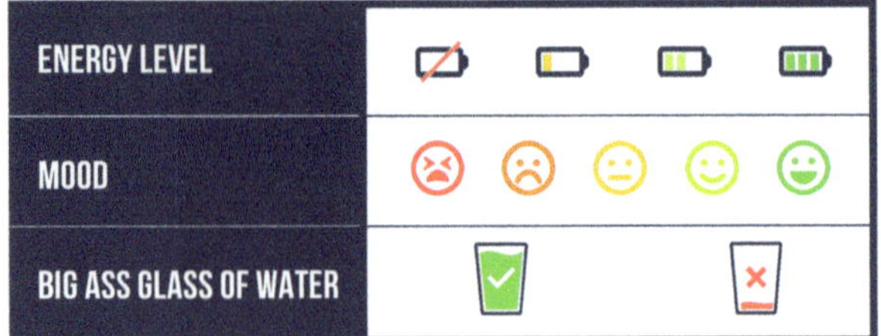

I AM GRATEFUL FOR:

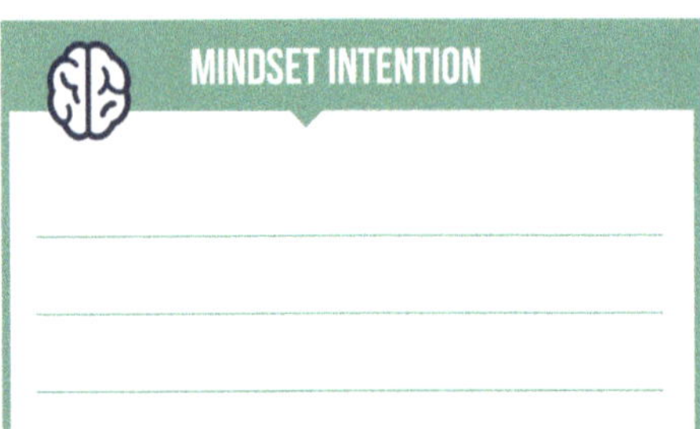

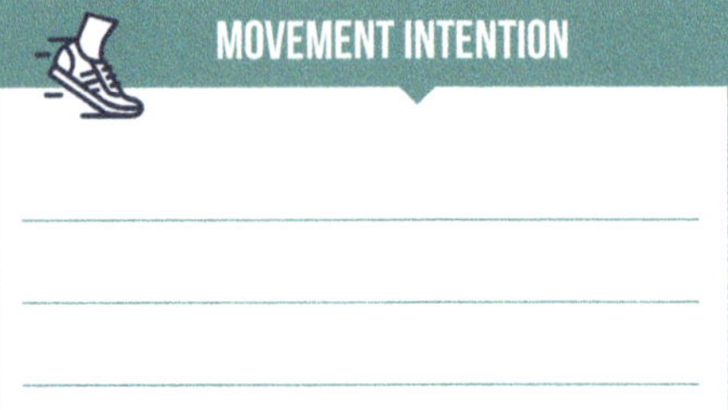

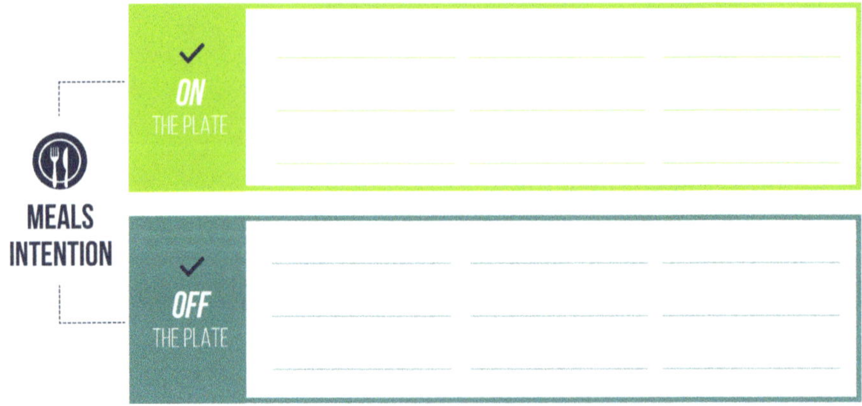

MINDFUL AFFIRMATION:

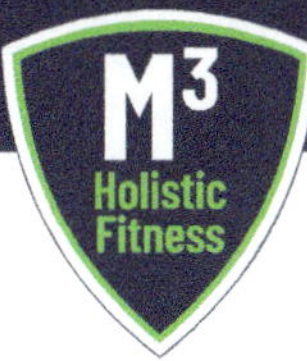

BEDTIME:

HYDRATION | 1 | 2 | 3 | 4 | 5 | 6 | 7 | 8 |

WHAT DIDN'T WORK TODAY?:

MOVEMENT: ☐

MEALS: ☐ ON ☐ OFF

TODAY'S WINS:

1

2

3

TODAY'S TAKE AWAY:

FOOD FOR THOUGHT FOR THE DAY:

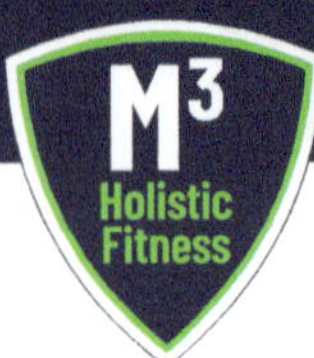

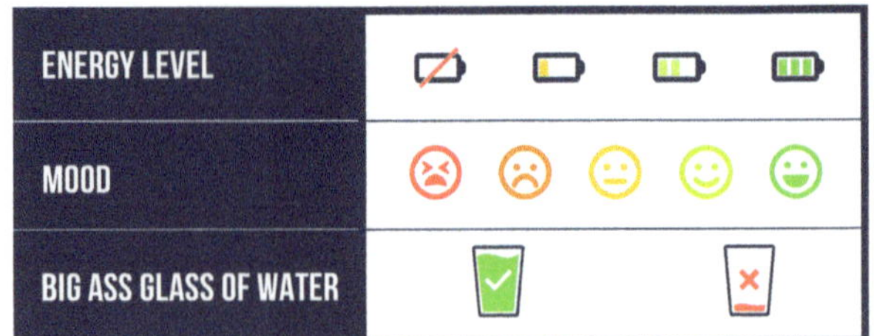

TODAYS DATE:

___ / ___ / ___

I AM GRATEFUL FOR:

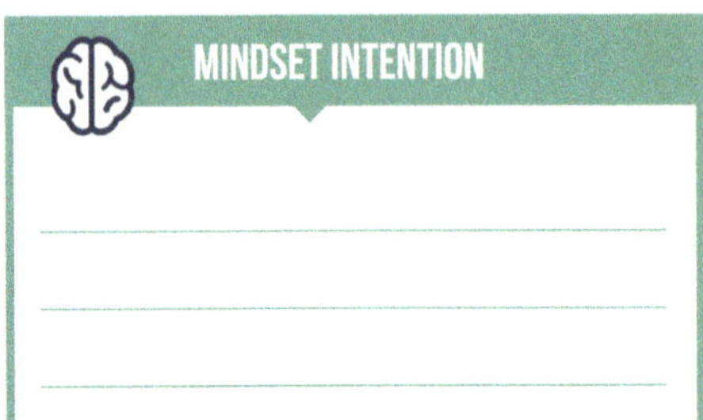

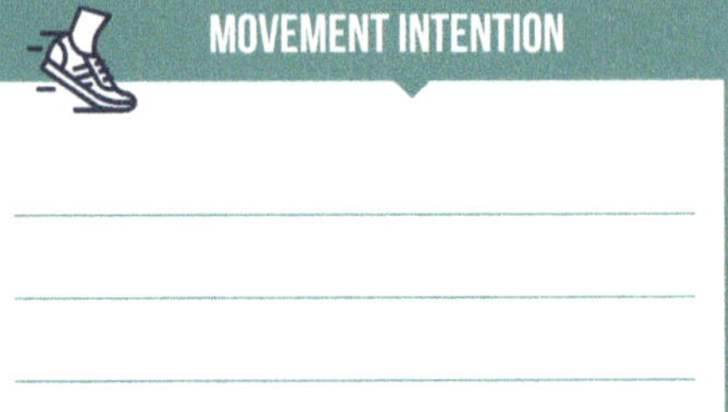

MINDFUL AFFIRMATION:

HYDRATION | 1 | 2 | 3 | 4 | 5 | 6 | 7 | 8 |

WHAT DIDN'T WORK TODAY?:

MOVEMENT: ☐

MEALS: ☐ ON ☐ OFF

TODAY'S WINS:

1

2

3

TODAY'S TAKE AWAY:

FOOD FOR THOUGHT FOR THE DAY:

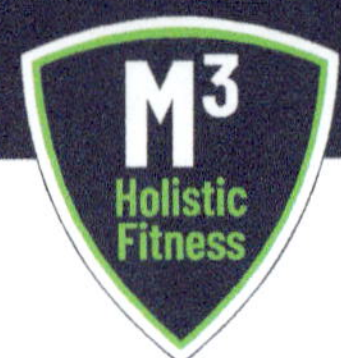

RISE AND ALIGN

WAKE UP: ____   SLEEP: ____ Hrs

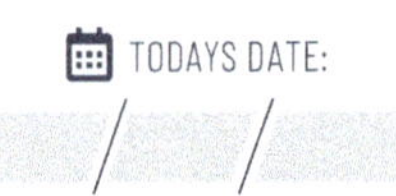

📅 TODAYS DATE: ____ / ____ / ____

ENERGY LEVEL				
MOOD				
BIG ASS GLASS OF WATER				

I AM GRATEFUL FOR:

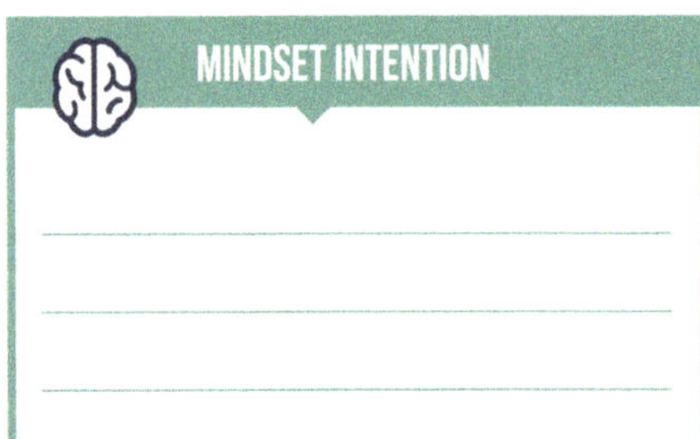

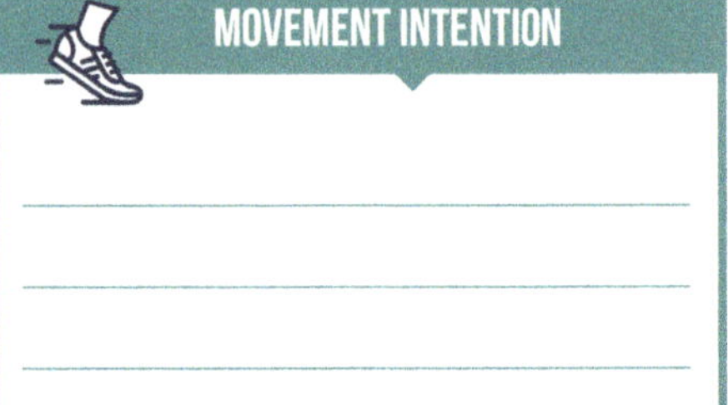

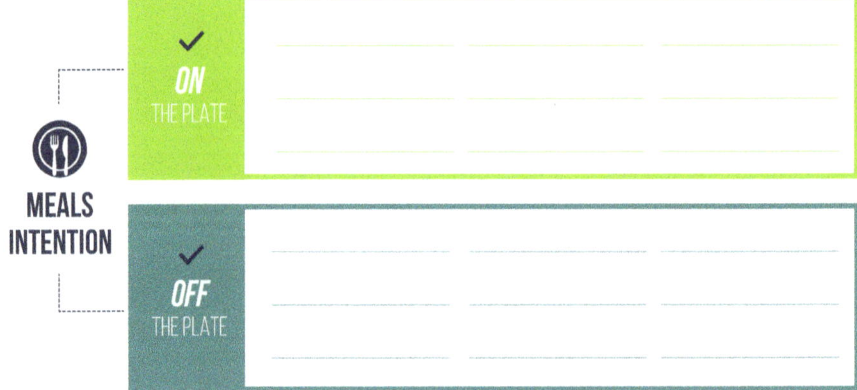

MINDFUL AFFIRMATION:

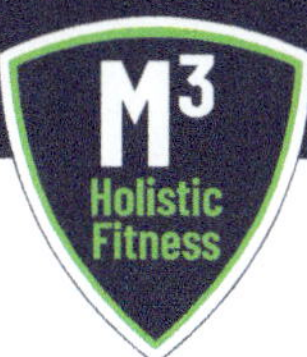

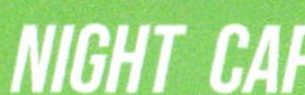

WHAT DIDN'T WORK TODAY?:

MOVEMENT:

MEALS:
ON   OFF

TODAY'S WINS:

1
2
3

TODAY'S TAKE AWAY:

FOOD FOR THOUGHT FOR THE DAY:

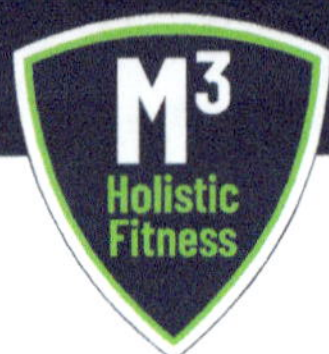

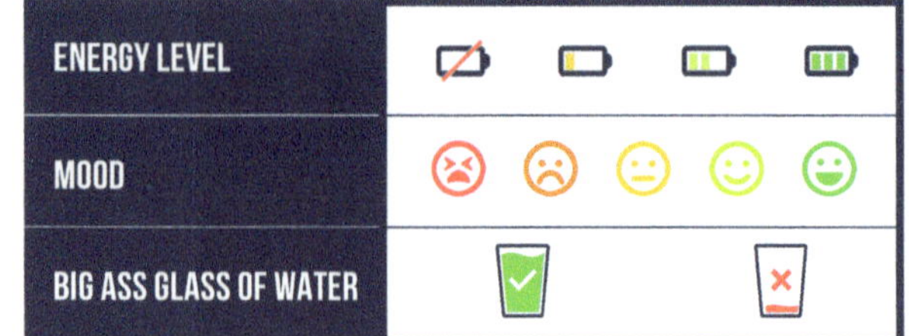

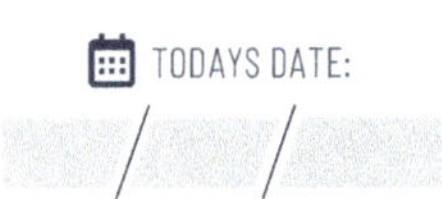

TODAYS DATE:

_____ / _____ / _____

ENERGY LEVEL				
MOOD				
BIG ASS GLASS OF WATER				

I AM GRATEFUL FOR:

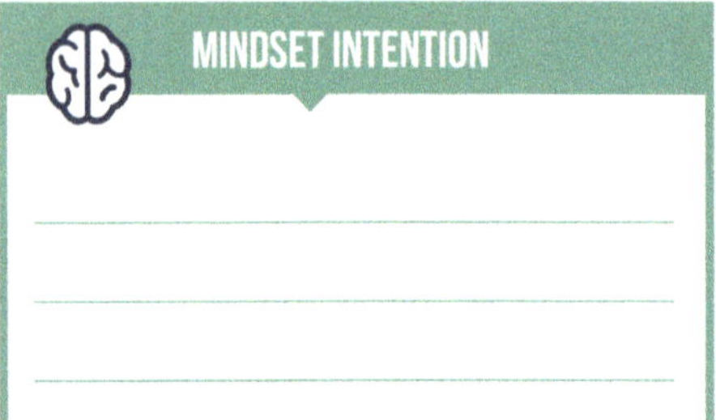

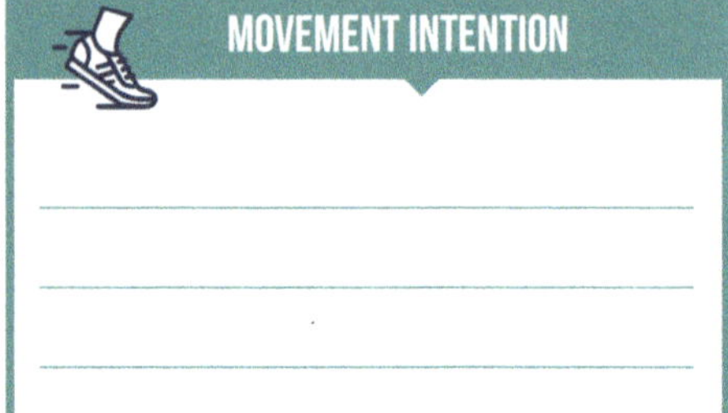

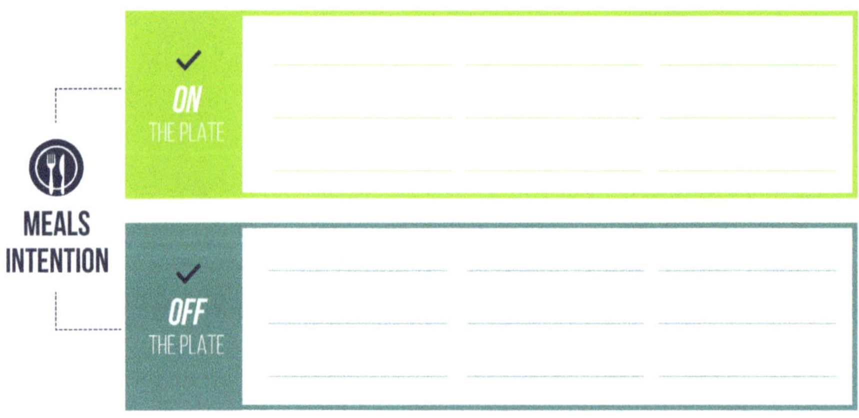

MEALS
INTENTION

MINDFUL AFFIRMATION:

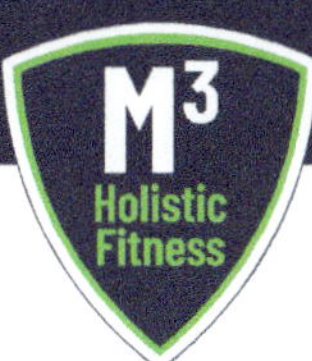

BEDTIME:

HYDRATION 1 2 3 4 5 6 7 8

WHAT DIDN'T WORK TODAY?:

MOVEMENT: ☐

MEALS: ☐ ON ☐ OFF

TODAY'S WINS: 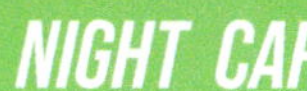

1

2

3

TODAY'S TAKE AWAY:

FOOD FOR THOUGHT FOR THE DAY:

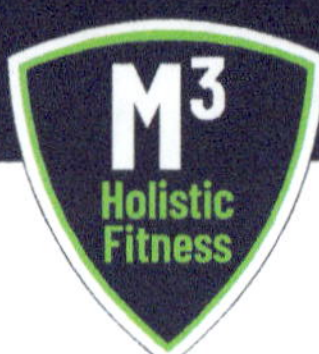

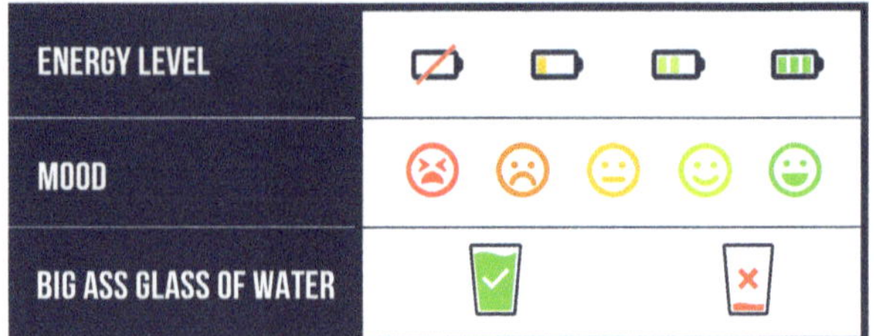

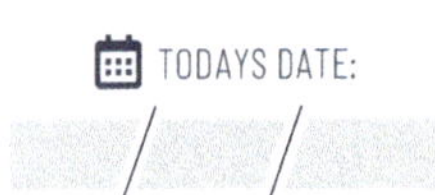
TODAYS DATE:
___ / ___ / ___

ENERGY LEVEL				
MOOD				
BIG ASS GLASS OF WATER				

I AM GRATEFUL FOR:

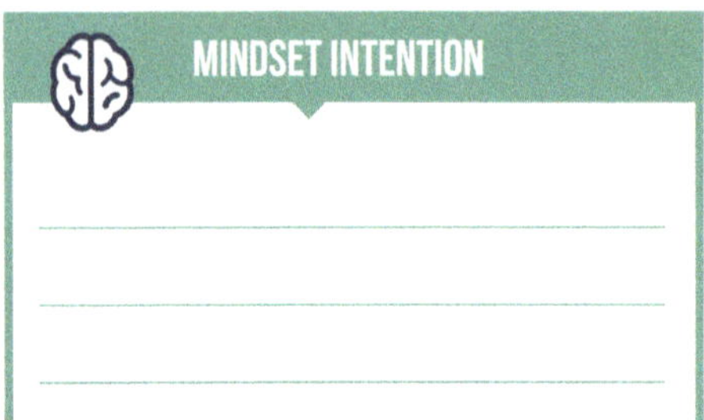

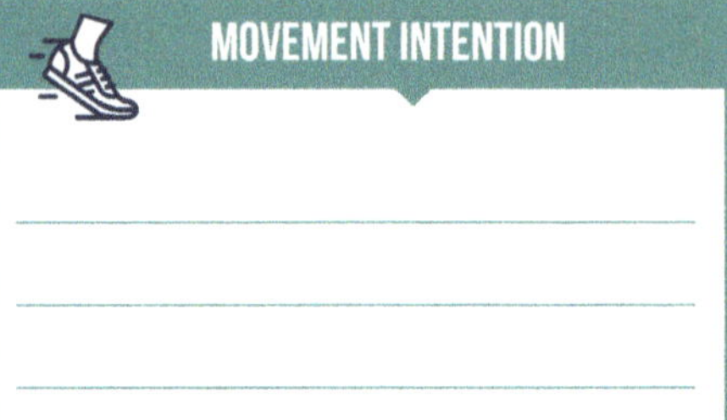

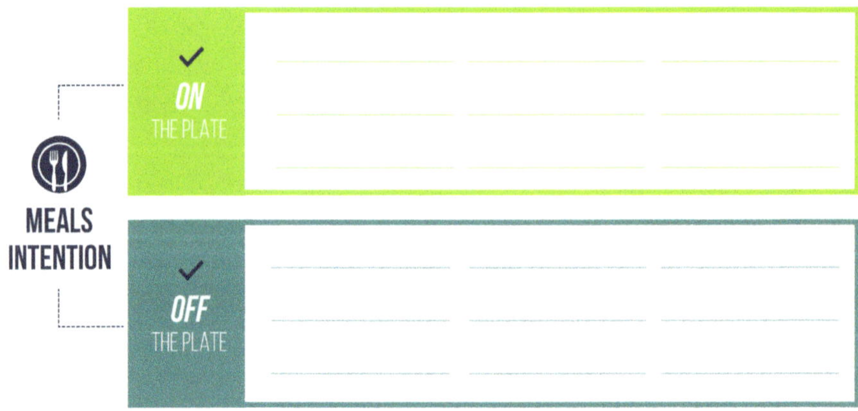

MINDFUL AFFIRMATION:

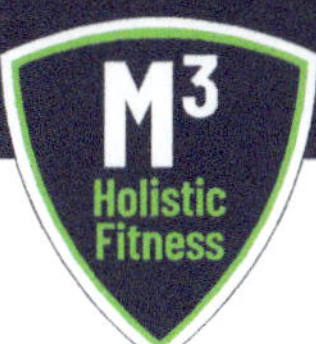

NIGHT CAP

BEDTIME:

HYDRATION   1 2 3 4 5 6 7 8

WHAT DIDN'T WORK TODAY?:

MOVEMENT:

MEALS: ON OFF

TODAY'S WINS: 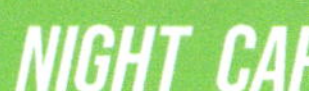

1

2

3

TODAY'S TAKE AWAY:

FOOD FOR THOUGHT FOR THE DAY:

66

At 211 degrees, water is hot.
At 212 degrees, it boils.
With boiling water comes steam, and with steam, you can power a train. One extra degree makes all the difference.

- 212 The Extra Degree

What is your extra degree?

Congratulations on completing 60 days of the Rise and Align Journal! You are in the process of creating a new way of being and living. Lean into what's working, and let go of what's not.

THE 60 DAYS IN REVIEW:

What are your top 3 wins from the past 60 days?

What have you learned about yourself additionally these past 30 days?

What are the M3 outcomes you want out of the next 30 days?
(Order your next Rise And Align 90–Day Journal…keep the momentum going.)

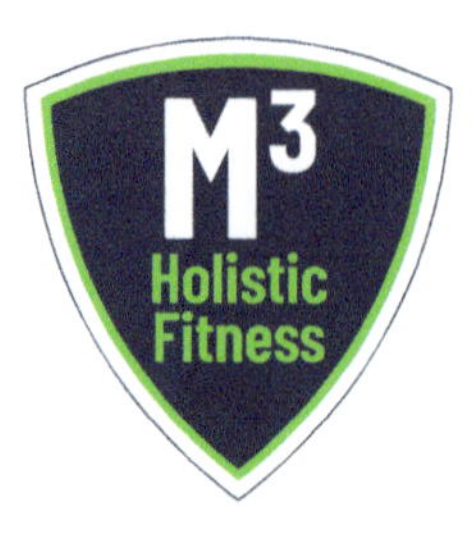

WEEK 9

90-DAY HOLISTIC FITNESS JOURNAL

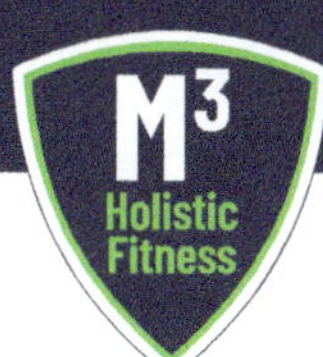

WHAT DOES YOUR LIFE LOOK LIKE?

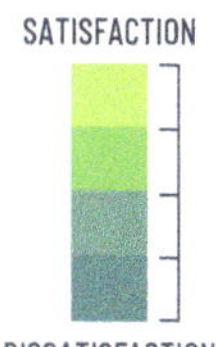

1. Place a dot in each category to indicate your level of satisfaction within each area. A dot at the **center of the circle to indicate dissatisfaction**, or towards the **outer edge to indicate satisfaction**. Most people fall somewhere in between. (see example)

2. Connect the dots to see your **M3 Circle of Life**.

3. Identify imbalances. Determine where to spend more time and energy to create balance. **This will help you create a better balance for your best Badass Life.**

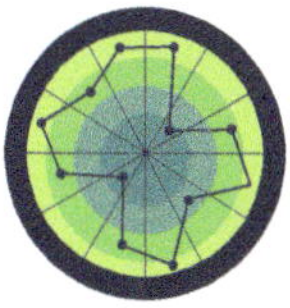

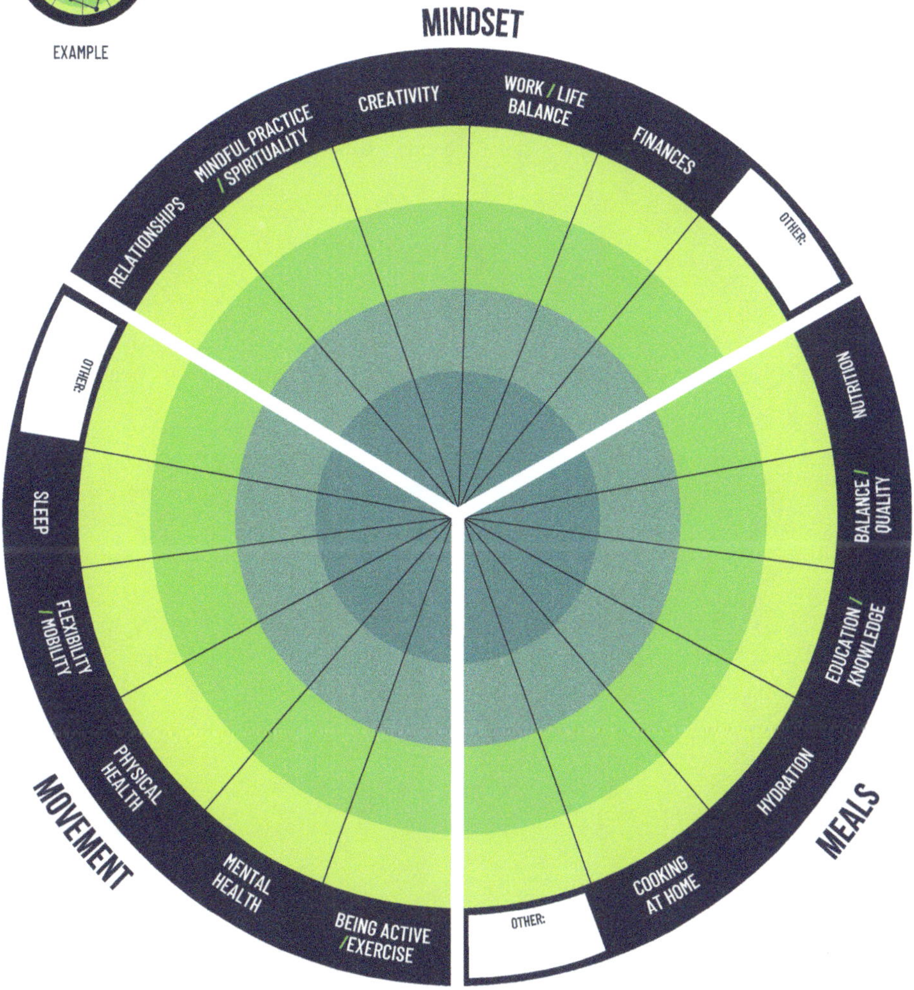

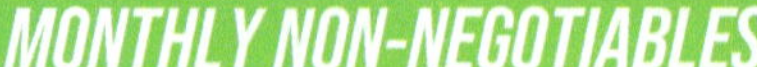
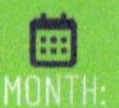

MONTH:

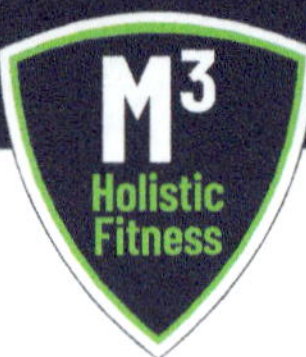

HABIT

DAY							
1							
2							
3							
4							
5							
6							
7							
8							
9							
10							
11							
12							
13							
14							
15							
16							
17							
18							
19							
20							
21							
22							
23							
24							
25							
26							
27							
28							
29							
30							
31							
TOTAL							

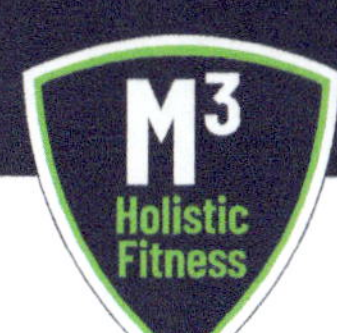

MAKE IT HAPPEN THIS WEEK

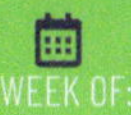

WEEK OF: ___ / ___ / ___

	MINDSET	MOVEMENT	MEALS	
			✓ ON THE PLATE	✓ OFF THE PLATE
MON				
TUES				
WEDS				
THURS				
FRI				
SAT				
SUN				

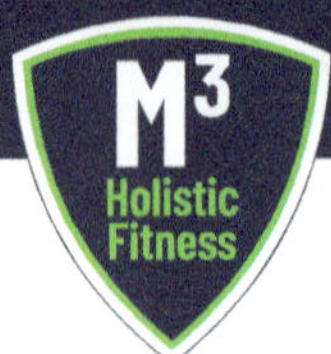

RISE AND ALIGN

WAKE UP: SLEEP: Hrs

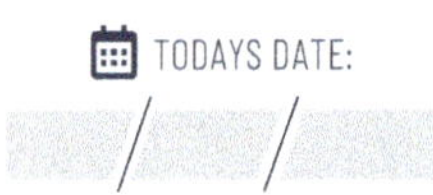

TODAYS DATE:

   /   /

ENERGY LEVEL				
MOOD				
BIG ASS GLASS OF WATER				

I AM GRATEFUL FOR:

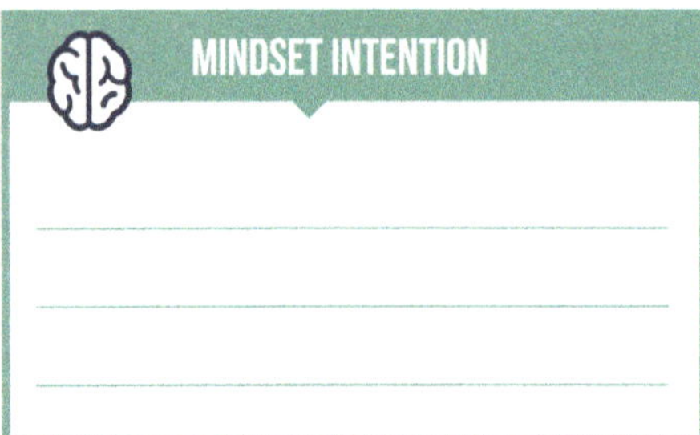

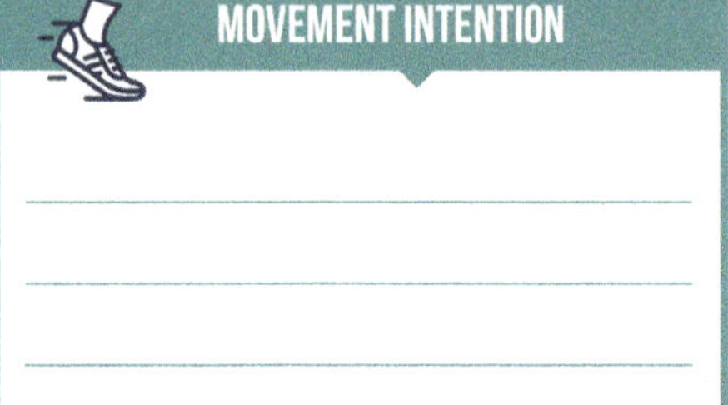

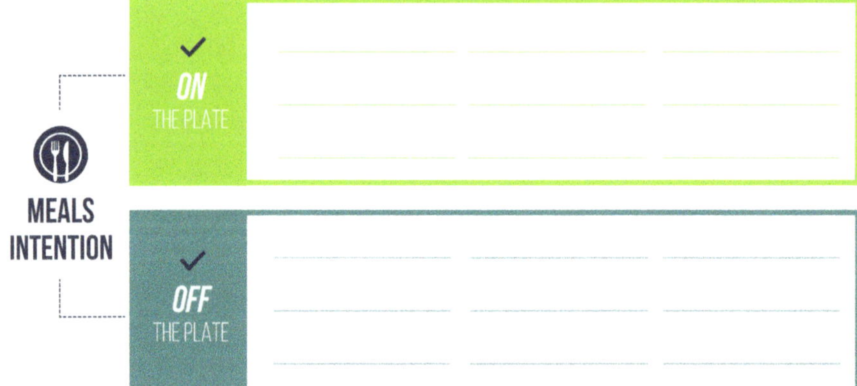

MINDFUL AFFIRMATION:

NIGHT CAP

BEDTIME:

HYDRATION 1 2 3 4 5 6 7 8

WHAT DIDN'T WORK TODAY?:

MOVEMENT: ☐

MEALS: ☐ ON ☐ OFF

TODAY'S WINS:

1

2

3

TODAY'S TAKE AWAY:

FOOD FOR THOUGHT FOR THE DAY:

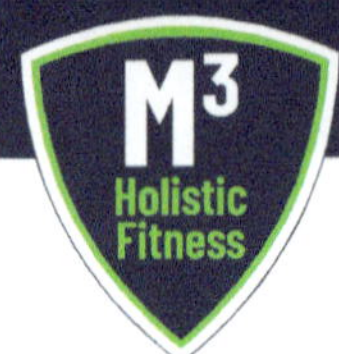

WAKE UP: SLEEP: Hrs

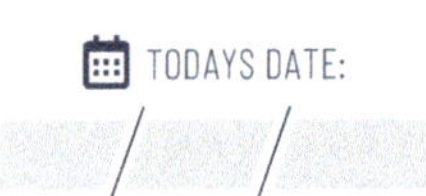

ENERGY LEVEL				
MOOD				
BIG ASS GLASS OF WATER				

I AM GRATEFUL FOR:

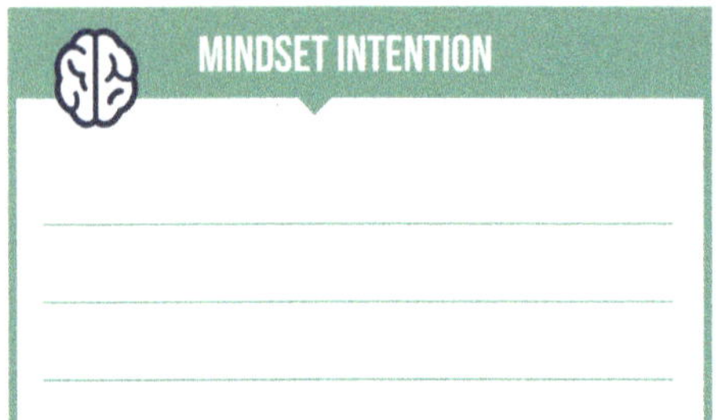

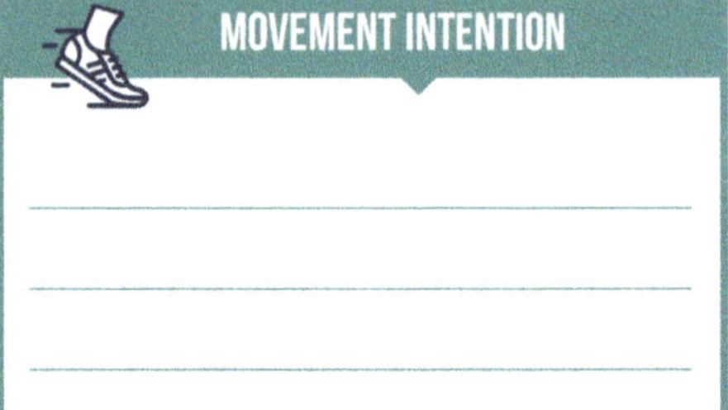

MINDFUL AFFIRMATION:

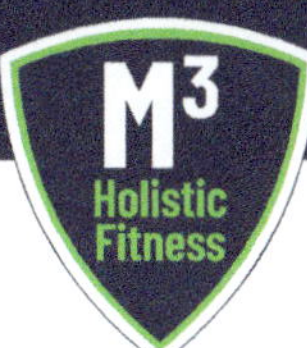

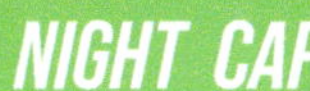

BEDTIME:

HYDRATION 1 2 3 4 5 6 7 8

WHAT DIDN'T WORK TODAY?:

MOVEMENT:

MEALS: ON OFF

TODAY'S WINS:

1

2

3

TODAY'S TAKE AWAY:

FOOD FOR THOUGHT FOR THE DAY:

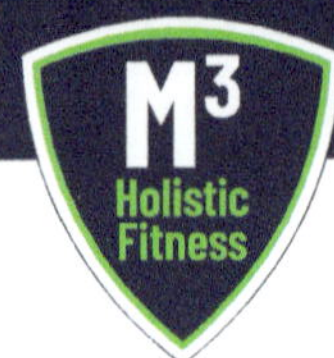

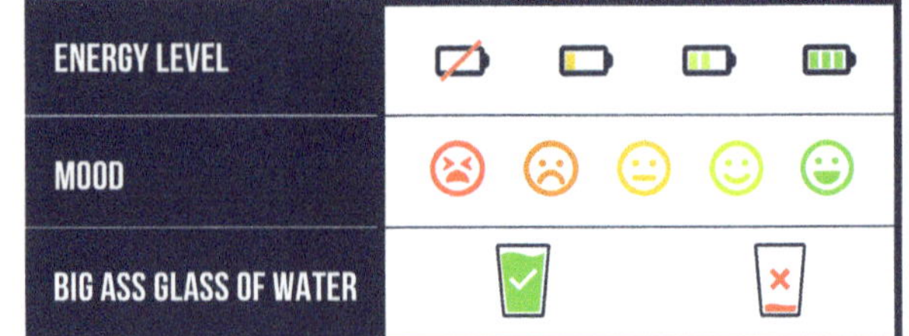

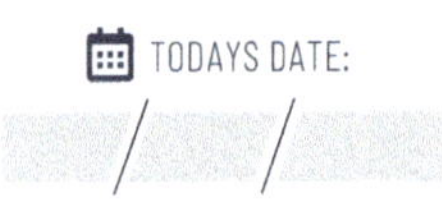

TODAYS DATE:

/ /

ENERGY LEVEL	
MOOD	
BIG ASS GLASS OF WATER	

I AM GRATEFUL FOR:

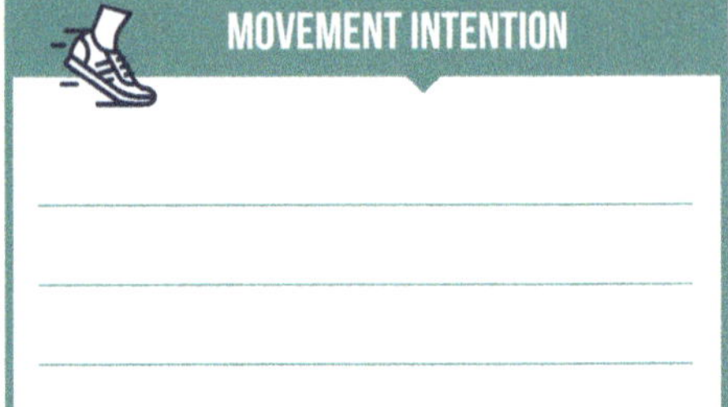

MINDFUL AFFIRMATION:

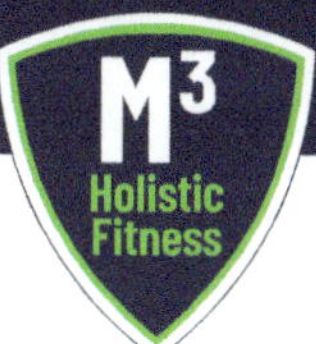

BEDTIME:

HYDRATION 1 2 3 4 5 6 7 8

WHAT DIDN'T WORK TODAY?:

MOVEMENT: ☐

MEALS: ☐ ON ☐ OFF

TODAY'S WINS: 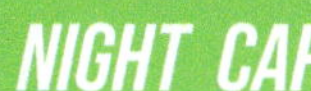

1

2

3

TODAY'S TAKE AWAY:

FOOD FOR THOUGHT FOR THE DAY:

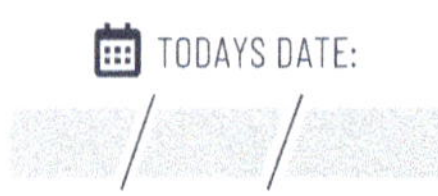 TODAYS DATE:
___ / ___ / ___

ENERGY LEVEL				
MOOD				
BIG ASS GLASS OF WATER				

I AM GRATEFUL FOR:

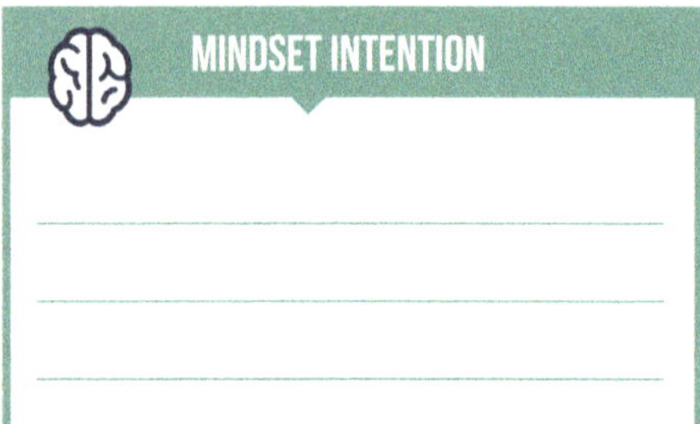

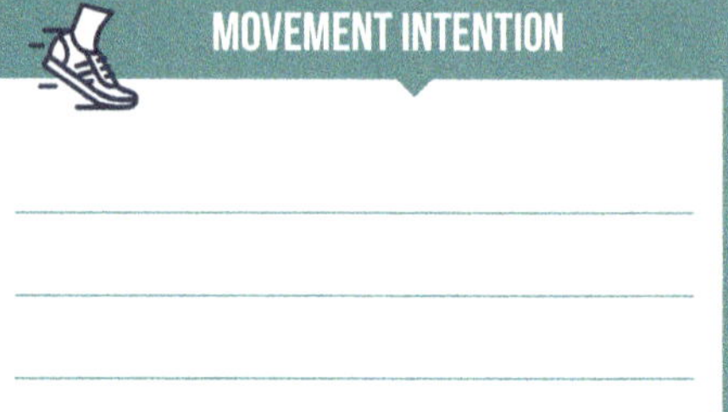

MEALS
INTENTION

MINDFUL AFFIRMATION:

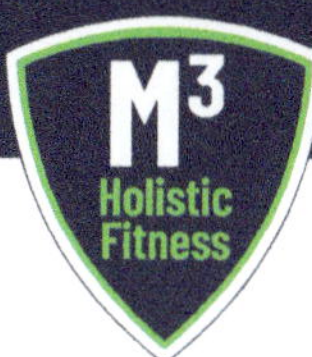

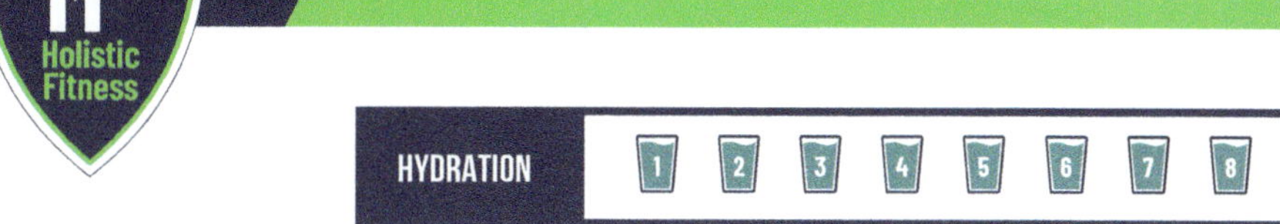

WHAT DIDN'T WORK TODAY?:

MOVEMENT: ☐

MEALS: ☐ ON ☐ OFF

TODAY'S WINS:

1

2

3

TODAY'S TAKE AWAY:

FOOD FOR THOUGHT FOR THE DAY:

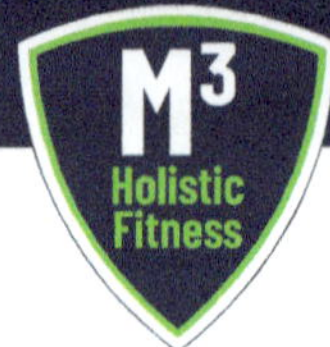

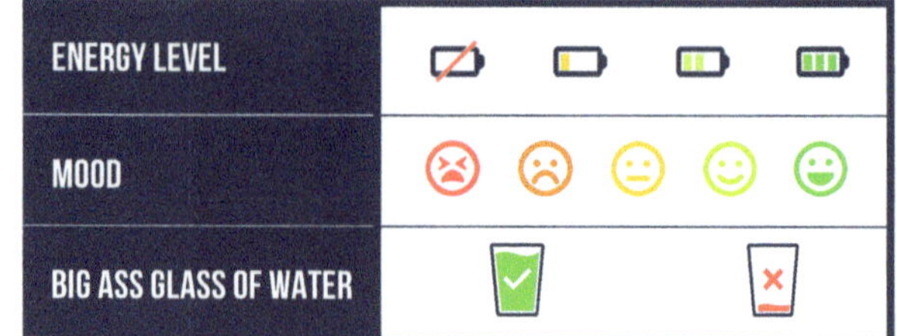

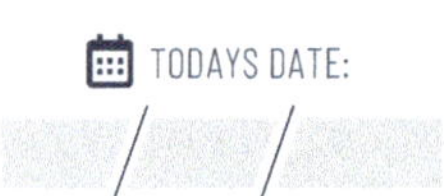

📅 TODAYS DATE:

_______ / _______ / _______

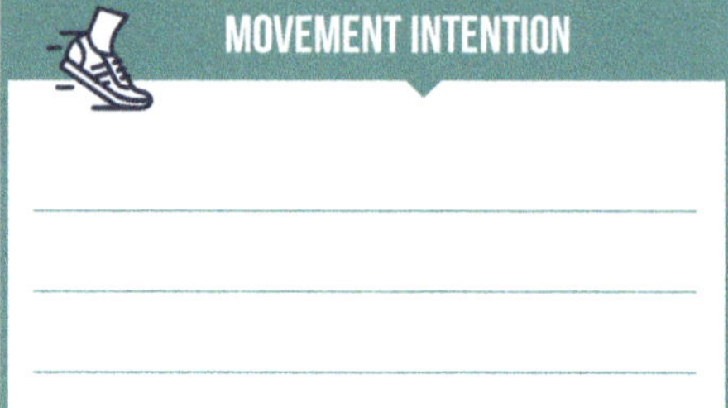

I AM GRATEFUL FOR:

MINDSET INTENTION	MOVEMENT INTENTION

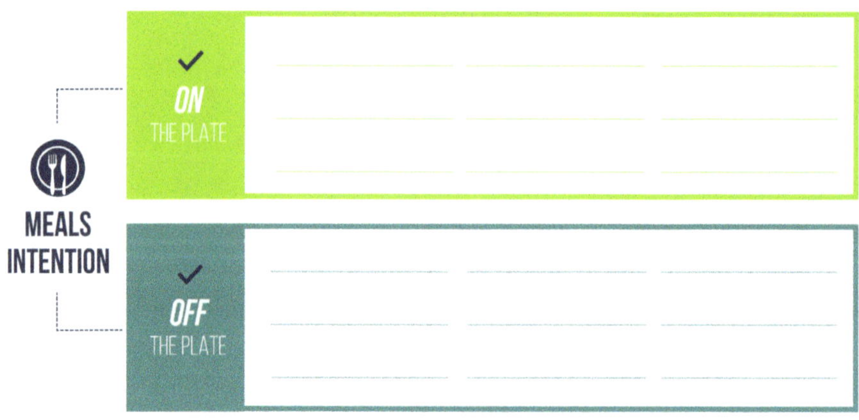

MINDFUL AFFIRMATION:

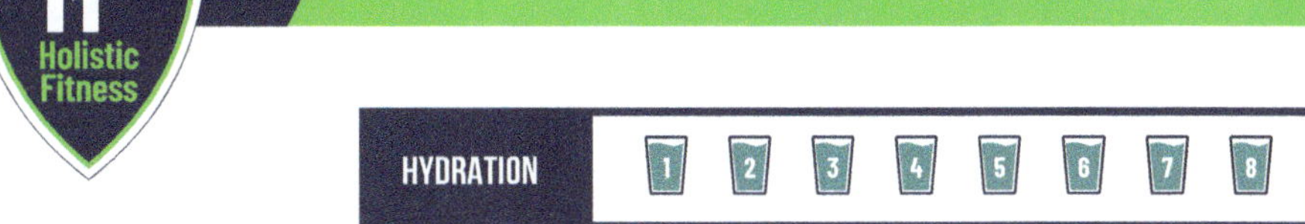

HYDRATION | 1 | 2 | 3 | 4 | 5 | 6 | 7 | 8

WHAT DIDN'T WORK TODAY?:

MOVEMENT: ☐

MEALS: ☐ ON ☐ OFF

TODAY'S WINS:

1

2

3

TODAY'S TAKE AWAY:

FOOD FOR THOUGHT FOR THE DAY:

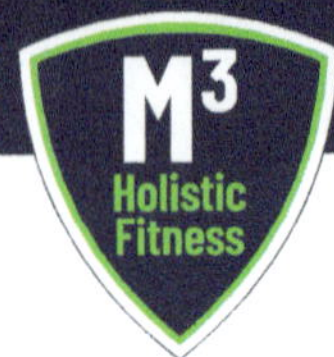

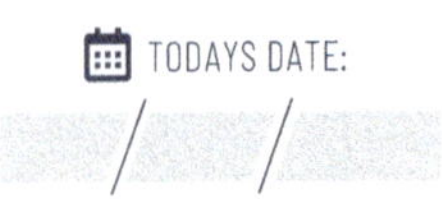

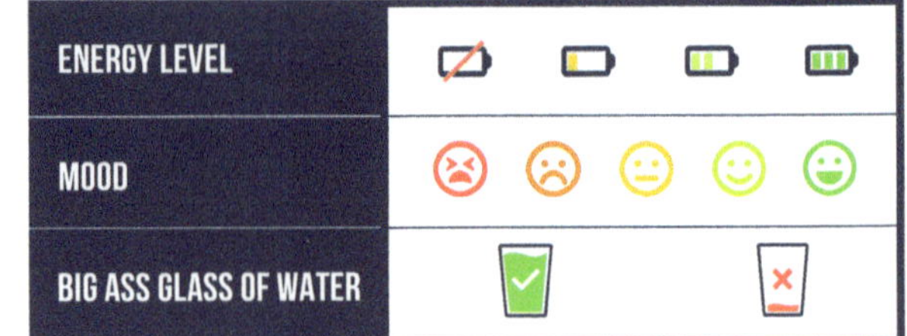

I AM GRATEFUL FOR:

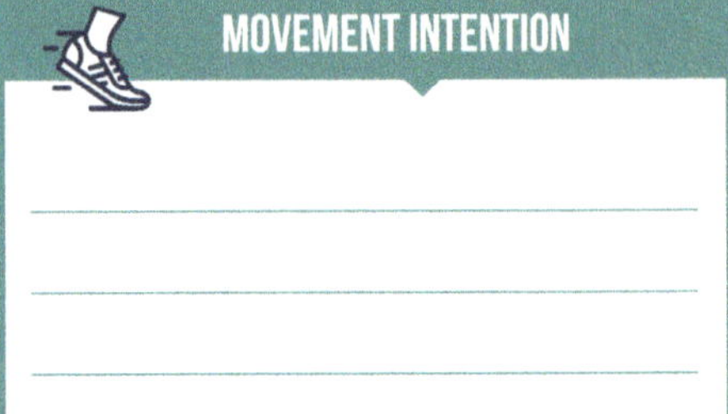

MINDFUL AFFIRMATION:

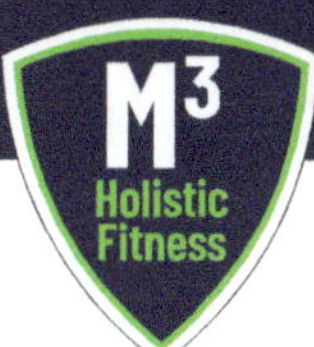

NIGHT CAP

BEDTIME:

HYDRATION | 1 | 2 | 3 | 4 | 5 | 6 | 7 | 8 |

WHAT DIDN'T WORK TODAY?:

MOVEMENT: ☐

MEALS: ☐ ON ☐ OFF

TODAY'S WINS: 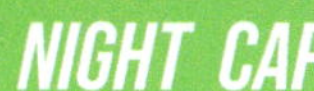

1

2

3

TODAY'S TAKE AWAY:

FOOD FOR THOUGHT FOR THE DAY:

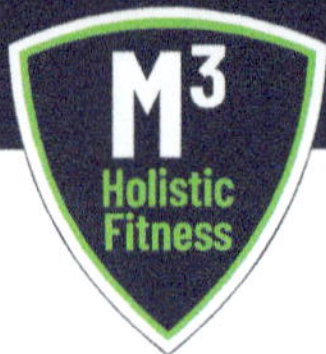

RISE AND ALIGN

WAKE UP: __________ SLEEP: ____ Hrs

ENERGY LEVEL	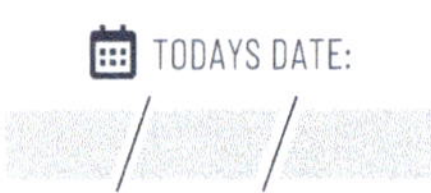
MOOD	
BIG ASS GLASS OF WATER	

TODAYS DATE: _____ / _____ / _____

I AM GRATEFUL FOR:

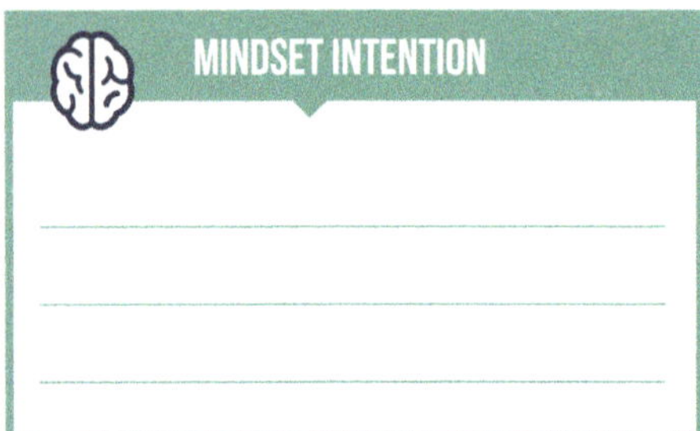

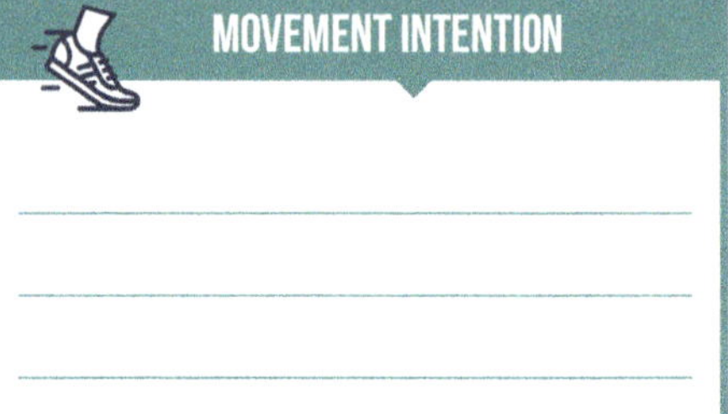

MEALS INTENTION

MINDFUL AFFIRMATION:

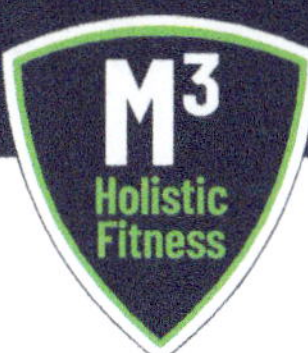

HYDRATION 1 2 3 4 5 6 7 8

WHAT DIDN'T WORK TODAY?:

MOVEMENT: ☐

MEALS: ☐ ON ☐ OFF

TODAY'S WINS: 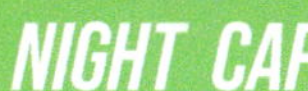

1

2

3

TODAY'S TAKE AWAY:

FOOD FOR THOUGHT FOR THE DAY:

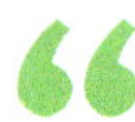

Doubt may be fatal to your dreams.

- My Dad

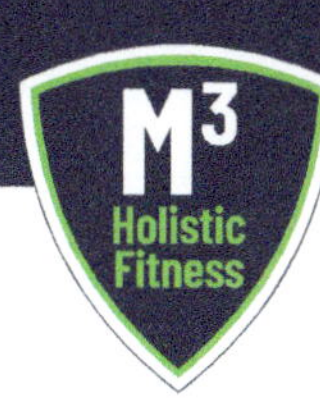

THIS WEEKS WINS:

THIS WEEKS TAKEAWAYS:

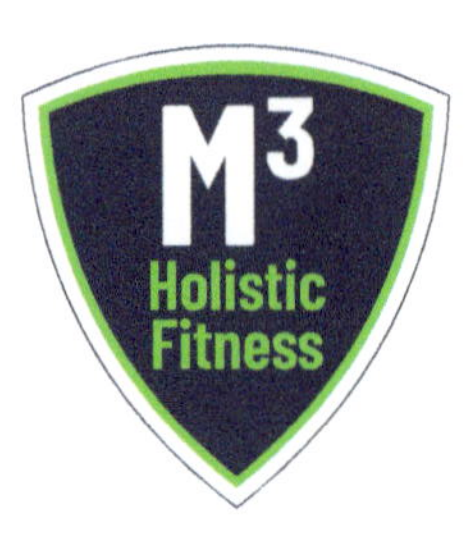

WEEK 10

90-DAY HOLISTIC FITNESS JOURNAL

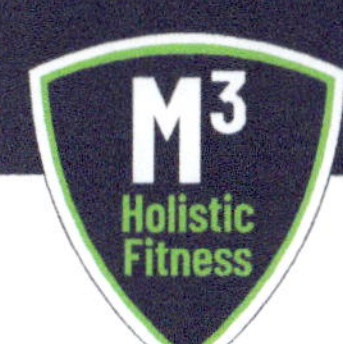

WHAT DOES YOUR LIFE LOOK LIKE?

1. Place a dot in each category to indicate your level of satisfaction within each area. A dot at the **center of the circle to indicate dissatisfaction**, or towards the **outer edge to indicate satisfaction**. Most people fall somewhere in between. (see example)

2. Connect the dots to see your M3 **Circle of Life**.

3. Identify imbalances. Determine where to spend more time and energy to create balance. **This will help you create a better balance for your best Badass Life.**

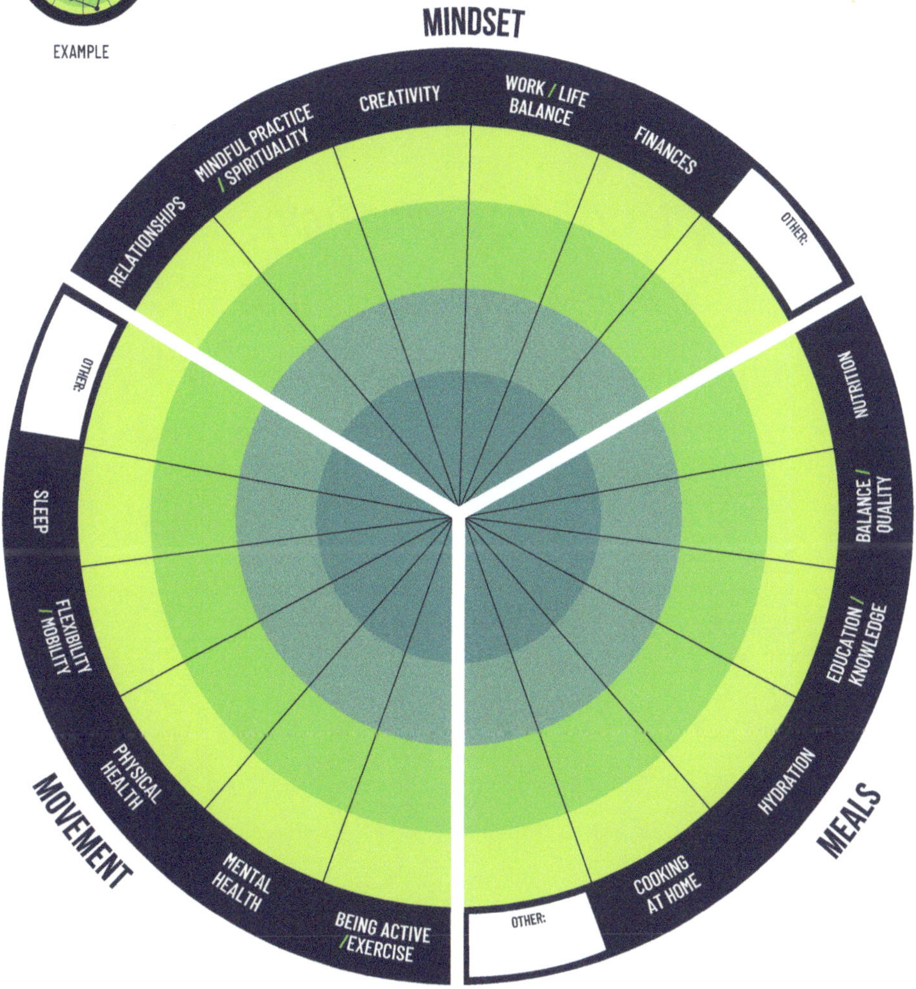

SATISFACTION

DISSATISFACTION

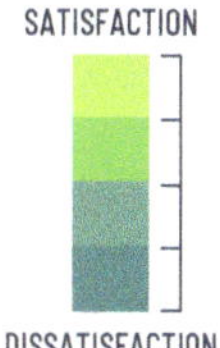

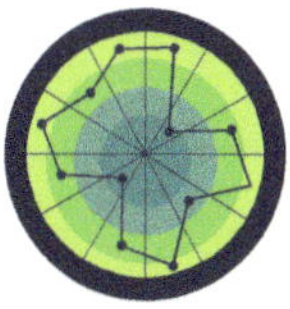

EXAMPLE

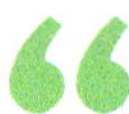

Good things come from change, and change comes from choice.

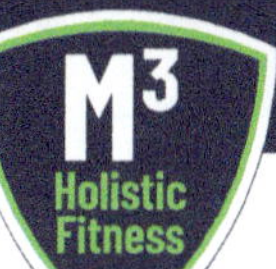

M³
Holistic Fitness

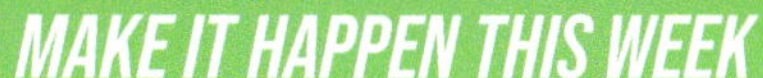

MAKE IT HAPPEN THIS WEEK

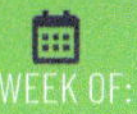

WEEK OF: ___/___/___

	MINDSET	MOVEMENT	MEALS	
			✓ ON THE PLATE	✓ OFF THE PLATE
MON				
TUES				
WEDS				
THURS				
FRI				
SAT				
SUN				

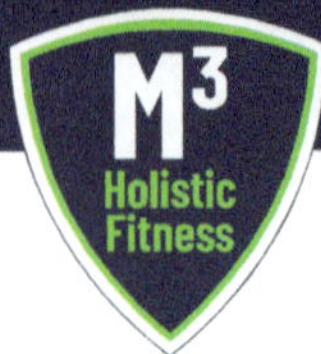

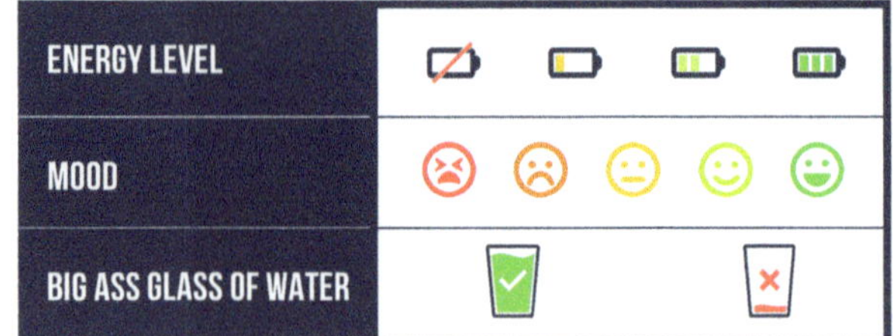

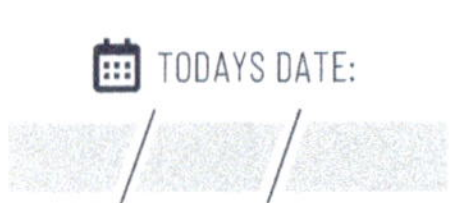

I AM GRATEFUL FOR:

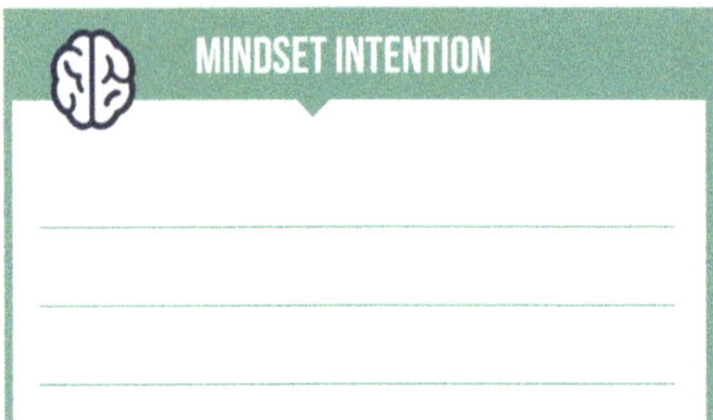

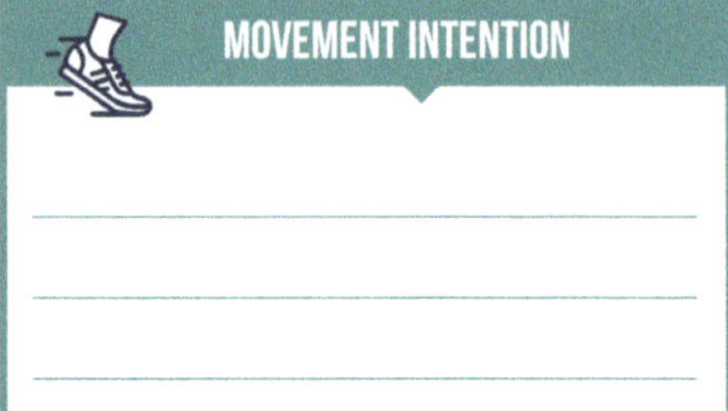

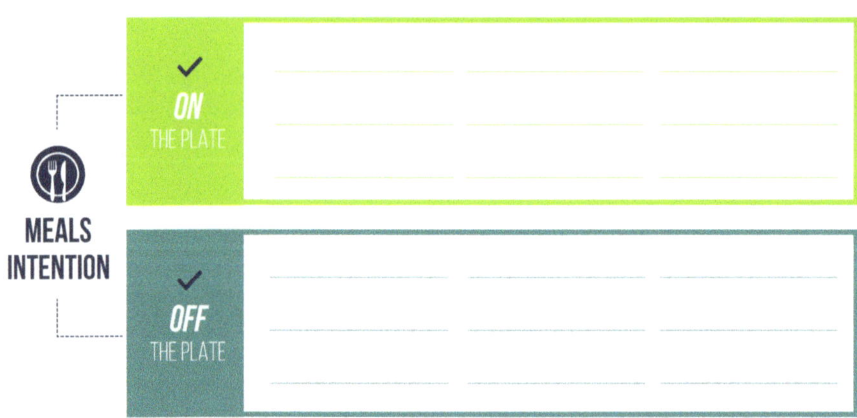

MINDFUL AFFIRMATION:

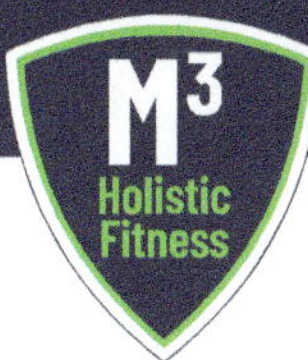

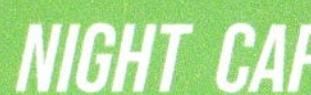
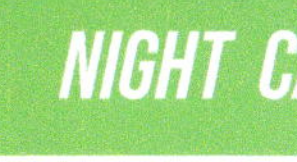
NIGHT CAP

WHAT DIDN'T WORK TODAY?:

MOVEMENT:

MEALS:

ON   OFF

TODAY'S WINS:

1

2

3

TODAY'S TAKE AWAY:

FOOD FOR THOUGHT FOR THE DAY:

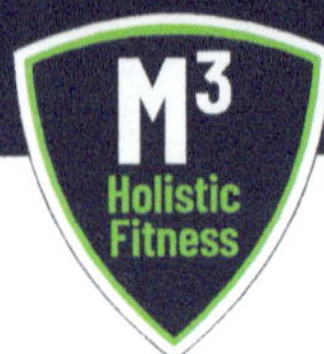

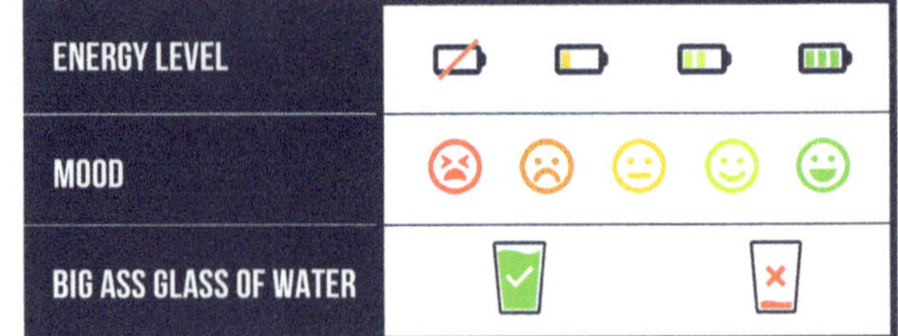

ENERGY LEVEL		
MOOD		
BIG ASS GLASS OF WATER		

I AM GRATEFUL FOR:

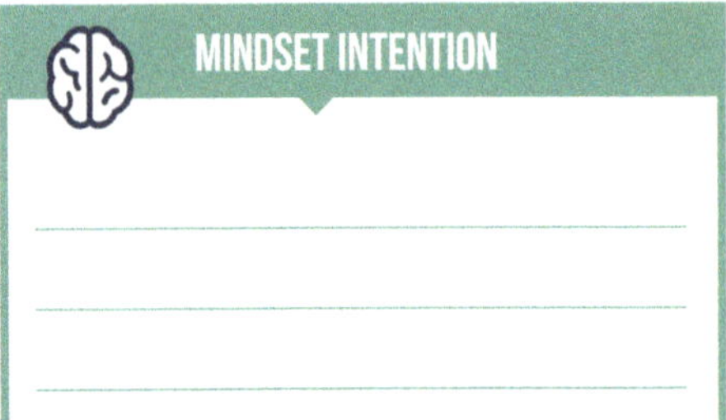

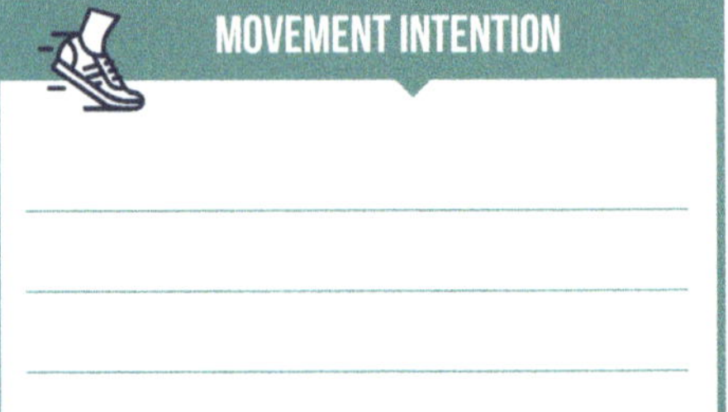

MINDFUL AFFIRMATION:

HYDRATION 1 2 3 4 5 6 7 8

WHAT DIDN'T WORK TODAY?:

MOVEMENT: ☐

MEALS: ☐ ON ☐ OFF

TODAY'S WINS:

1

2

3

TODAY'S TAKE AWAY:

FOOD FOR THOUGHT FOR THE DAY:

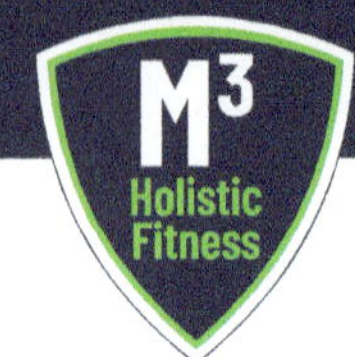

M³
Holistic Fitness

WAKE UP: ____________ SLEEP: ______ Hrs

ENERGY LEVEL				
MOOD				
BIG ASS GLASS OF WATER				

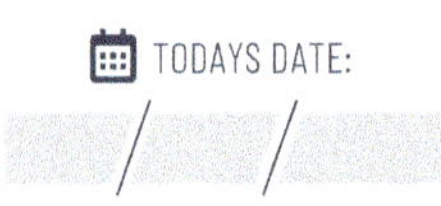

📅 TODAYS DATE: _____ / _____ / _____

I AM GRATEFUL FOR:

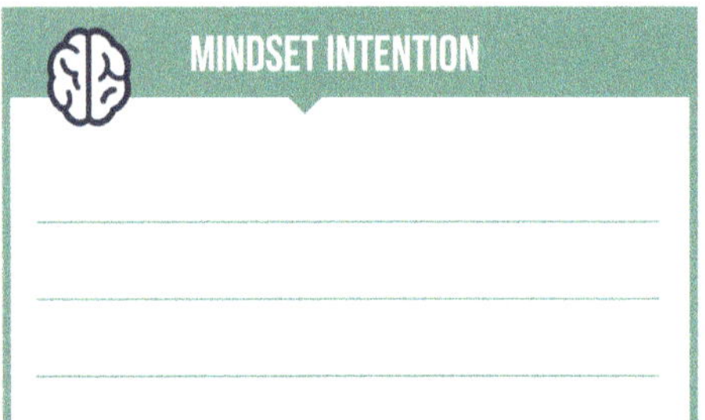

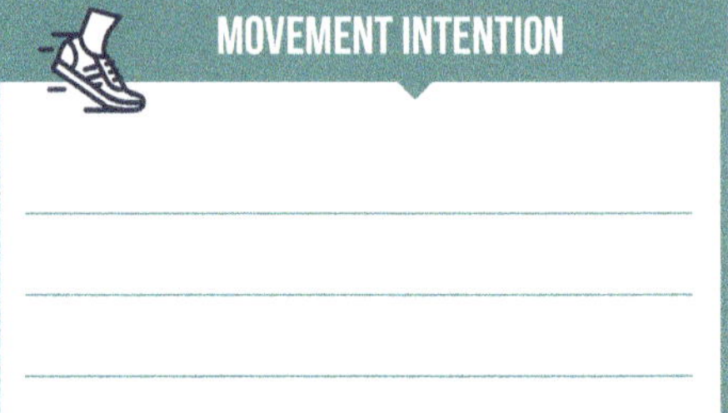

MEALS INTENTION

MINDFUL AFFIRMATION:

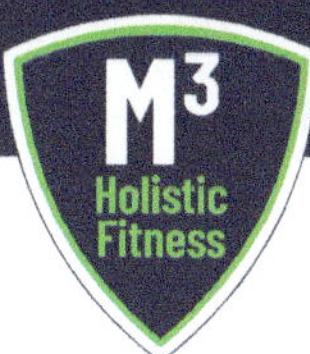

HYDRATION 1 2 3 4 5 6 7 8

WHAT DIDN'T WORK TODAY?:

MOVEMENT: ☐

MEALS: ☐ ON ☐ OFF

TODAY'S WINS: 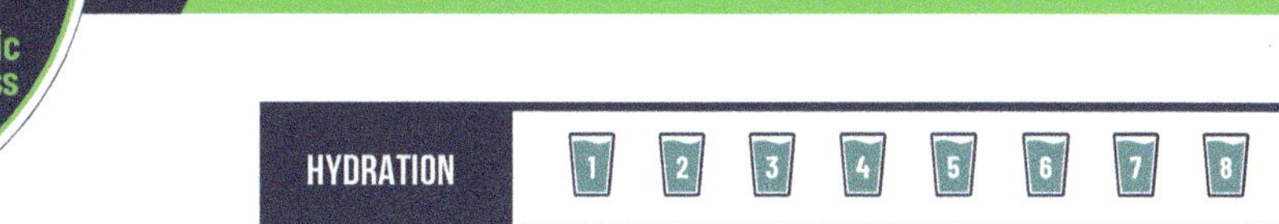

1

2

3

TODAY'S TAKE AWAY:

FOOD FOR THOUGHT FOR THE DAY:

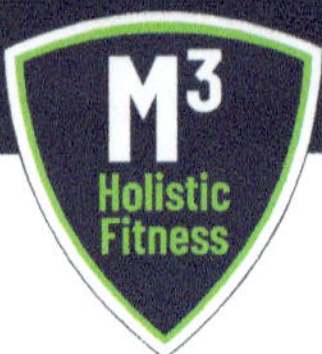

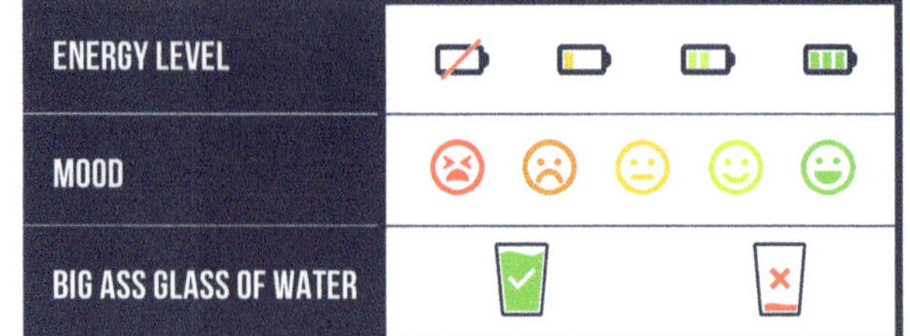

ENERGY LEVEL				
MOOD				
BIG ASS GLASS OF WATER				

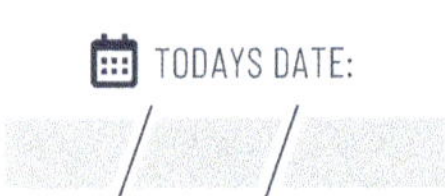

TODAYS DATE:

______ / ______ / ______

I AM GRATEFUL FOR:

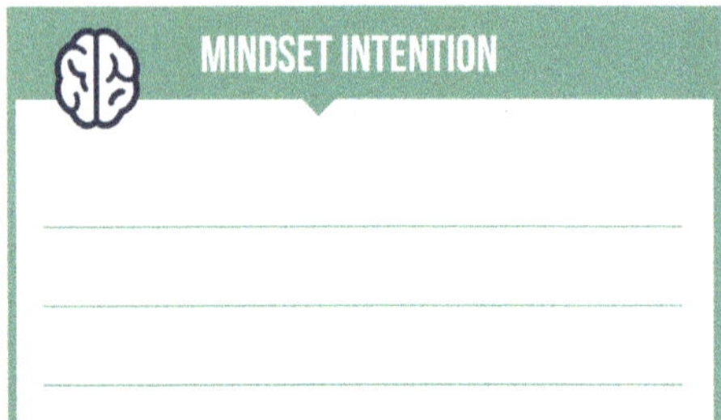

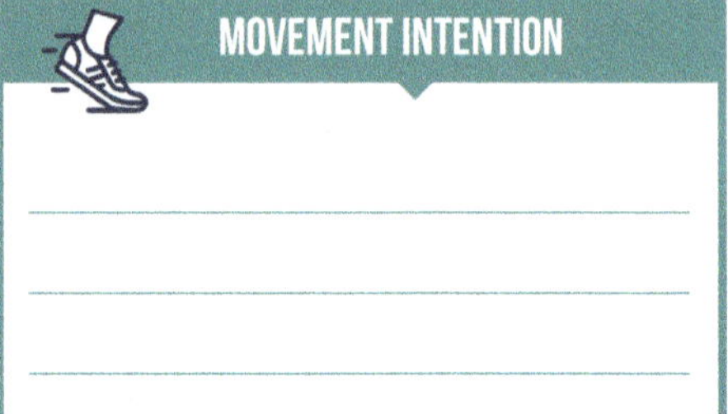

MINDFUL AFFIRMATION:

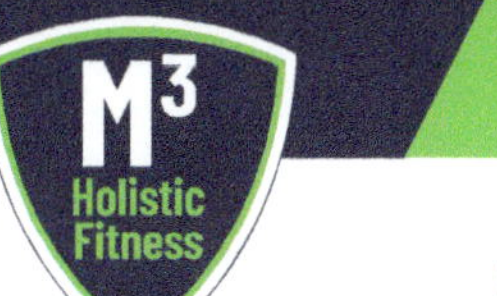

M³
Holistic Fitness

BEDTIME:

HYDRATION | 1 | 2 | 3 | 4 | 5 | 6 | 7 | 8

WHAT DIDN'T WORK TODAY?:

MOVEMENT: ☐

MEALS: ☐ ON ☐ OFF

TODAY'S WINS:

1

2

3

TODAY'S TAKE AWAY:

FOOD FOR THOUGHT FOR THE DAY:

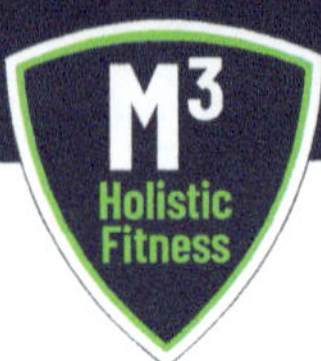

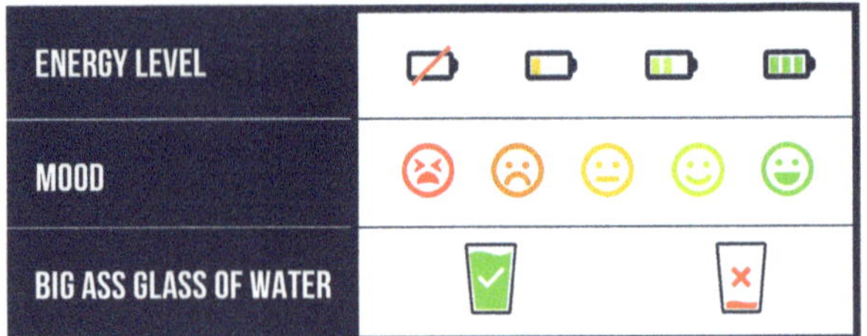

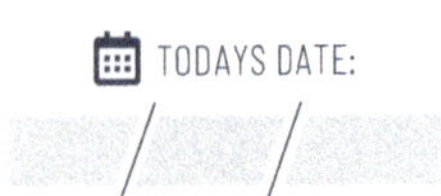

ENERGY LEVEL				
MOOD				
BIG ASS GLASS OF WATER				

I AM GRATEFUL FOR:

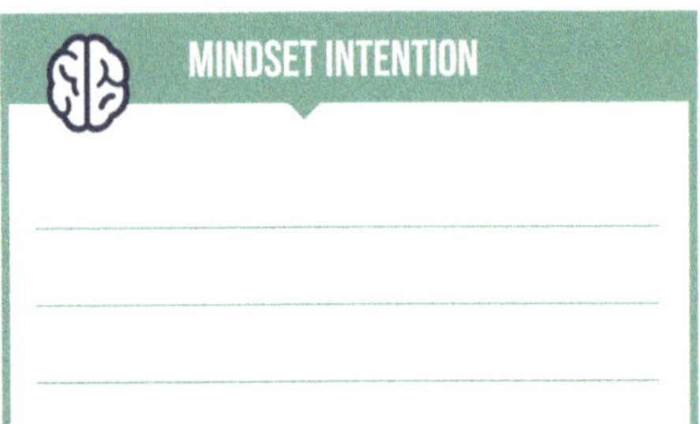

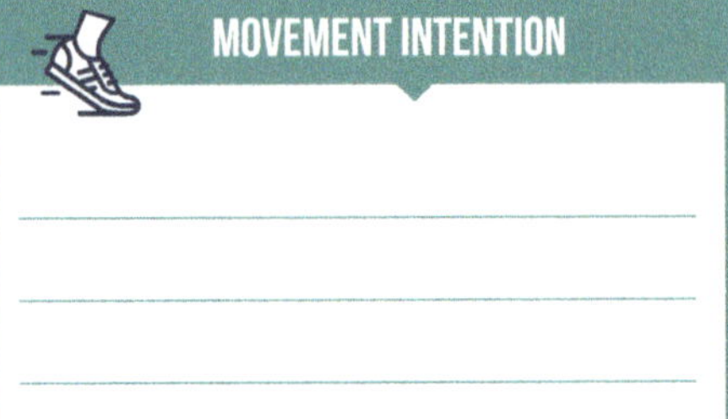

MEALS INTENTION

MINDFUL AFFIRMATION:

HYDRATION 1 2 3 4 5 6 7 8

WHAT DIDN'T WORK TODAY?:

MOVEMENT: □

MEALS: □ ON □ OFF

TODAY'S WINS:

1

2

3

TODAY'S TAKE AWAY:

FOOD FOR THOUGHT FOR THE DAY:

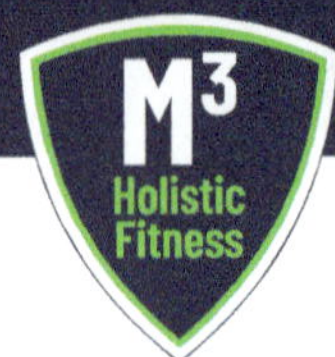
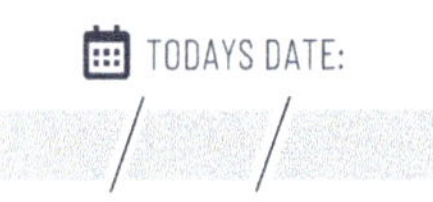

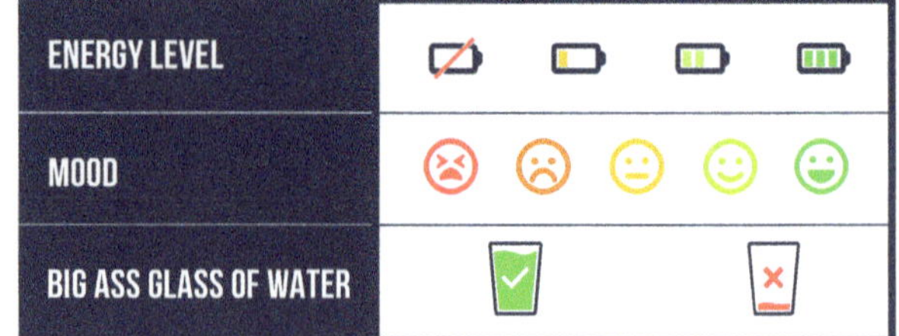

TODAYS DATE: ___ / ___ / ___

I AM GRATEFUL FOR:

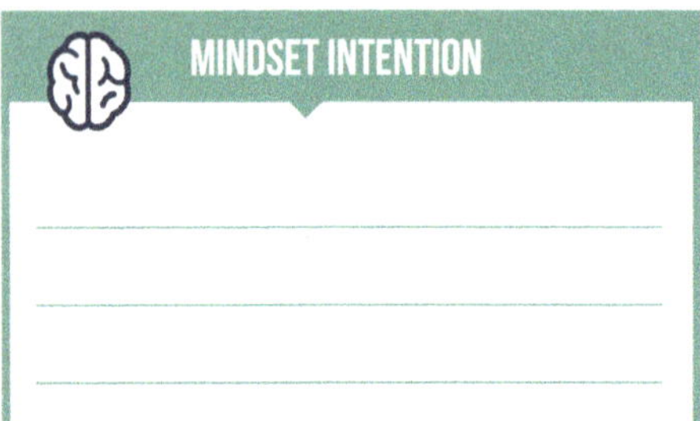

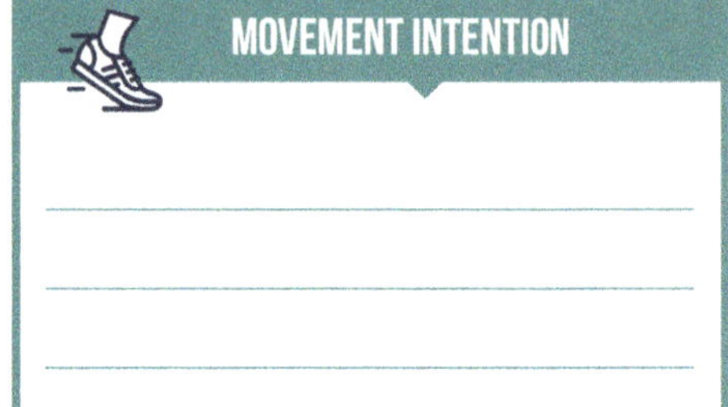

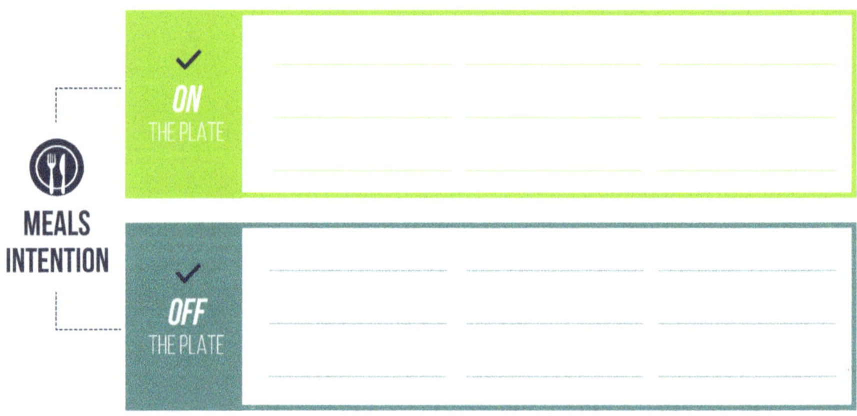

MINDFUL AFFIRMATION:

HYDRATION 1 2 3 4 5 6 7 8

WHAT DIDN'T WORK TODAY?:

MOVEMENT:

MEALS: ON OFF

TODAY'S WINS:

1

2

3

TODAY'S TAKE AWAY:

FOOD FOR THOUGHT FOR THE DAY:

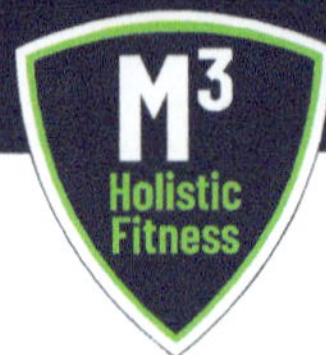

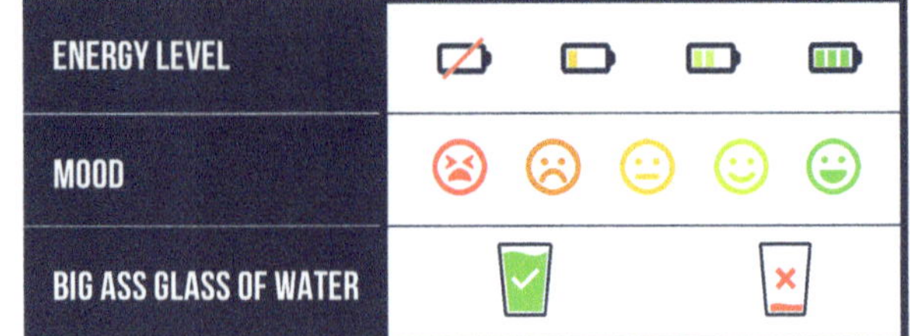

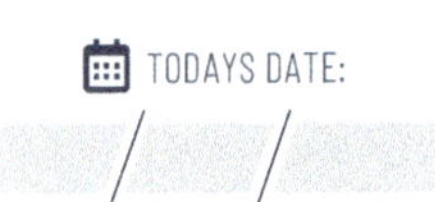

I AM GRATEFUL FOR:

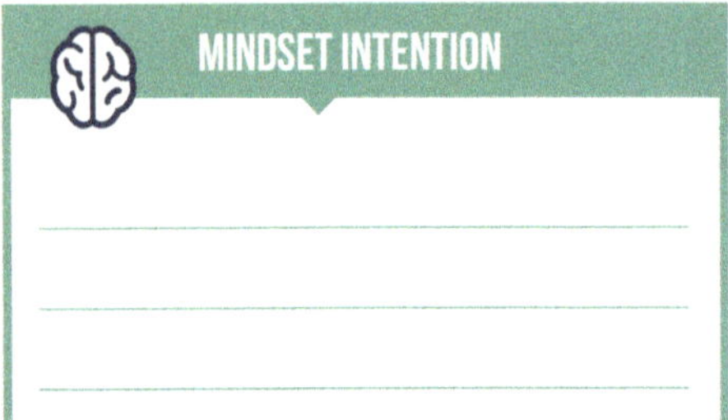

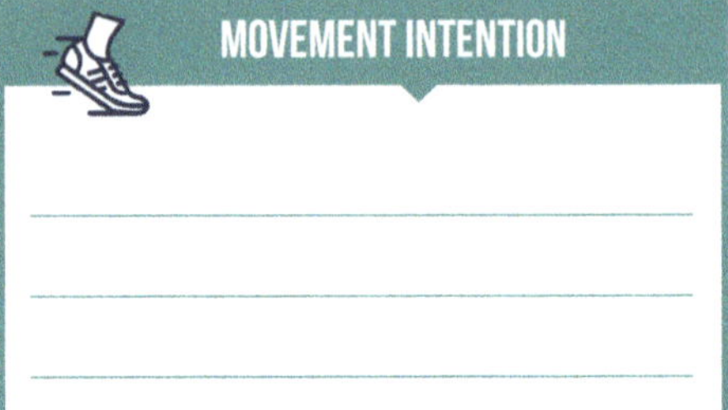

MINDFUL AFFIRMATION:

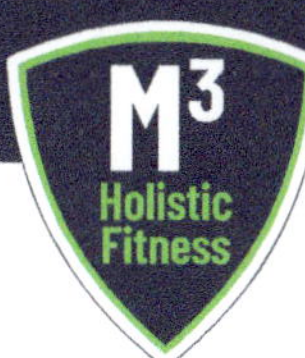

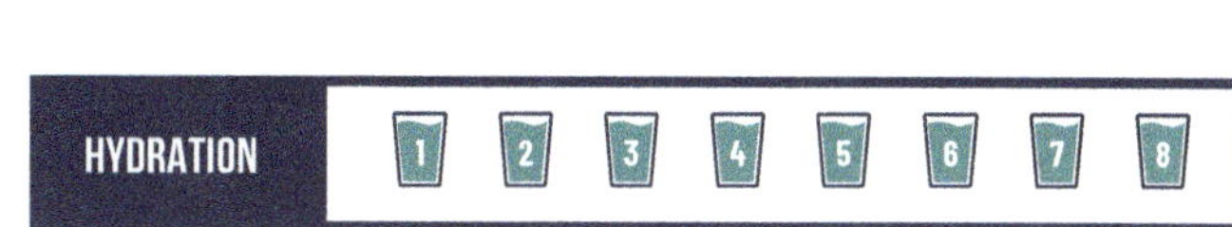

WHAT DIDN'T WORK TODAY?:

MOVEMENT:

MEALS:
ON   OFF

TODAY'S WINS:

1

2

3

TODAY'S TAKE AWAY:

FOOD FOR THOUGHT FOR THE DAY:

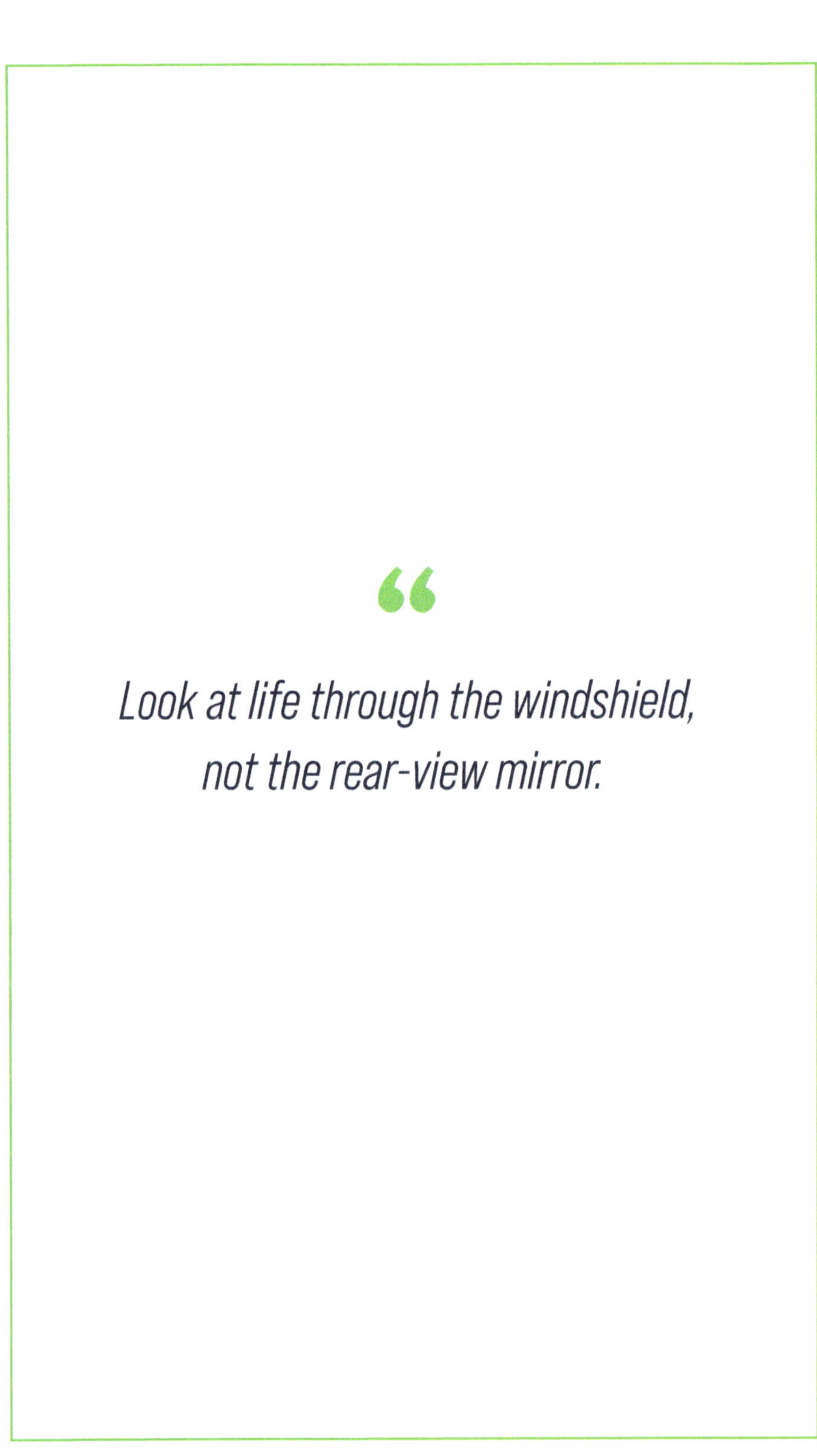

Look at life through the windshield,
not the rear-view mirror.

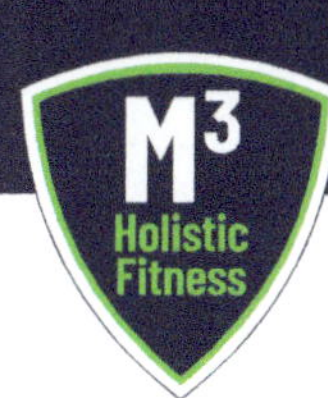

THIS WEEKS WINS:

THIS WEEKS TAKEAWAYS:

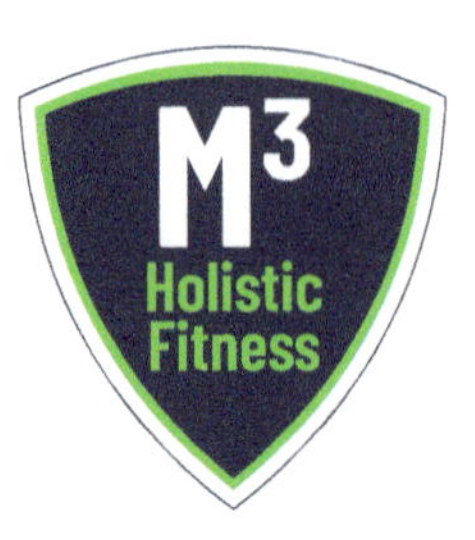

WEEK 11

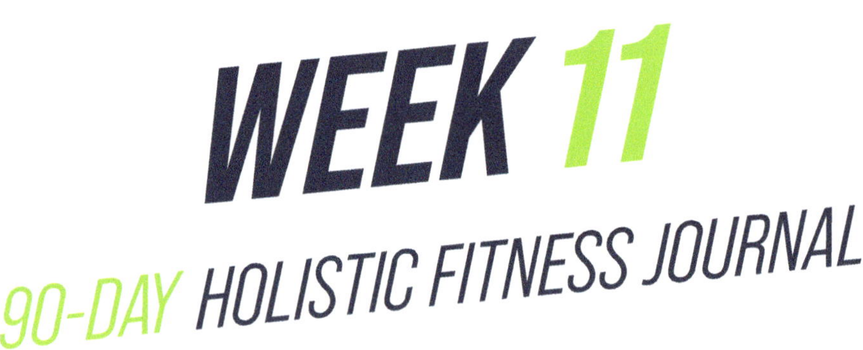

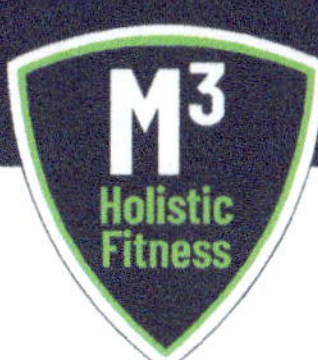

WHAT DOES YOUR LIFE LOOK LIKE?

SATISFACTION

DISSATISFACTION

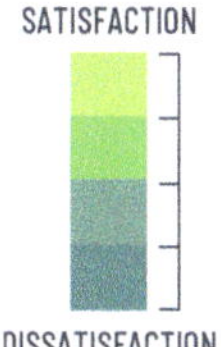

1. Place a dot in each category to indicate your level of satisfaction within each area. A dot at the **center of the circle to indicate dissatisfaction**, or towards the **outer edge to indicate satisfaction**. Most people fall somewhere in between. (see example)

2. Connect the dots to see your **M3 Circle of Life.**

3. Identify imbalances. Determine where to spend more time and energy to create balance. **This will help you create a better balance for your best Badass Life.**

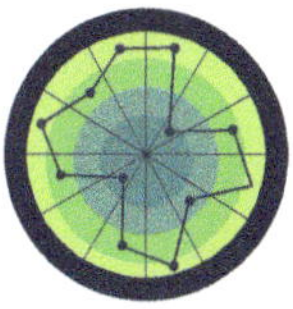

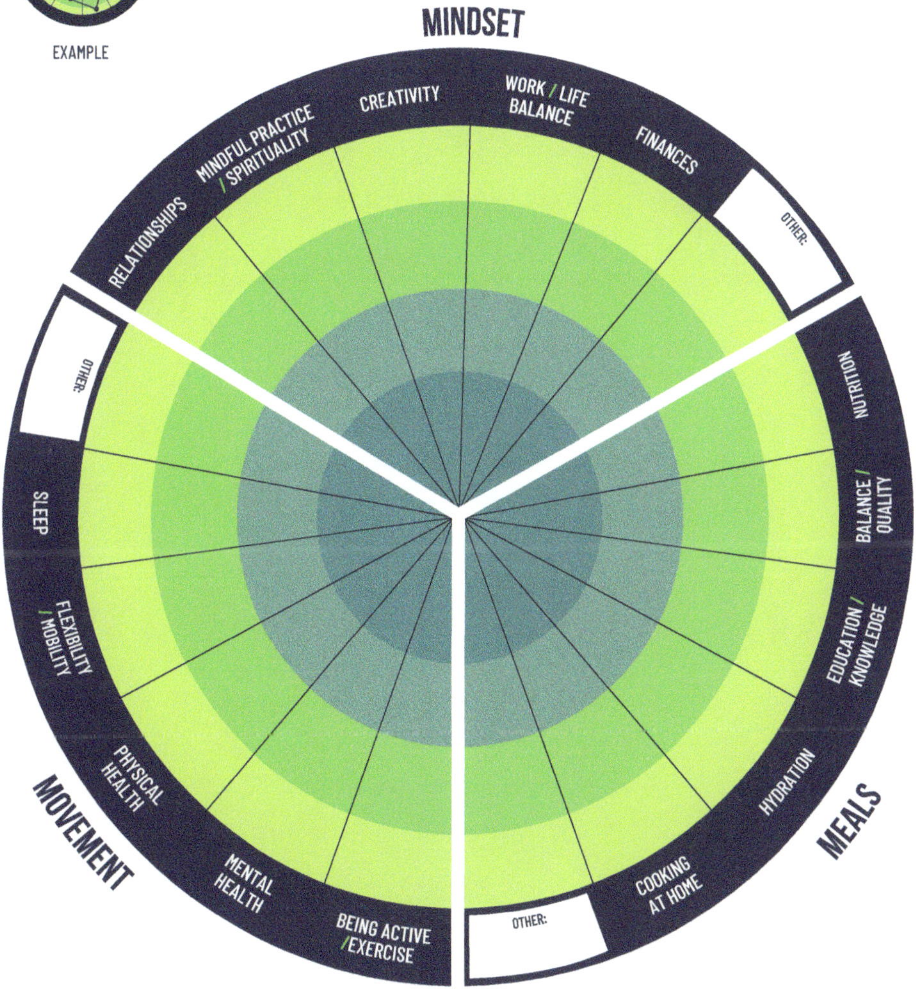

"

Instead of worrying about what you cannot control, shift your energy to what you can create.

	MINDSET	MOVEMENT	MEALS ✓ ON THE PLATE	MEALS ✓ OFF THE PLATE
MON				
TUES				
WEDS				
THURS				
FRI				
SAT				
SUN				

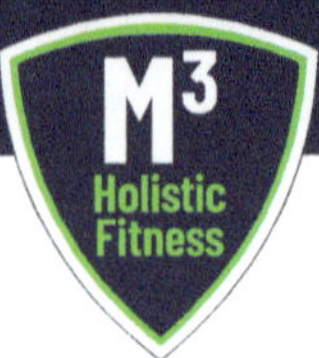

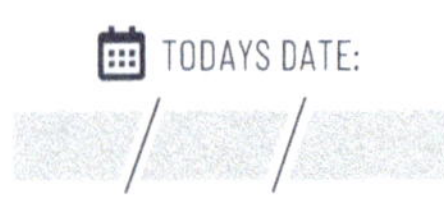

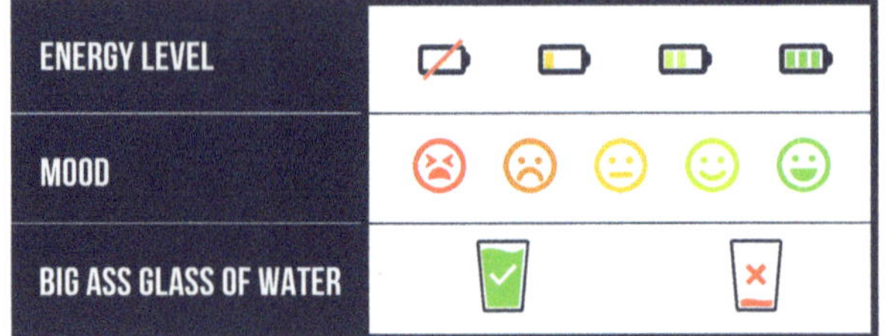

I AM GRATEFUL FOR:

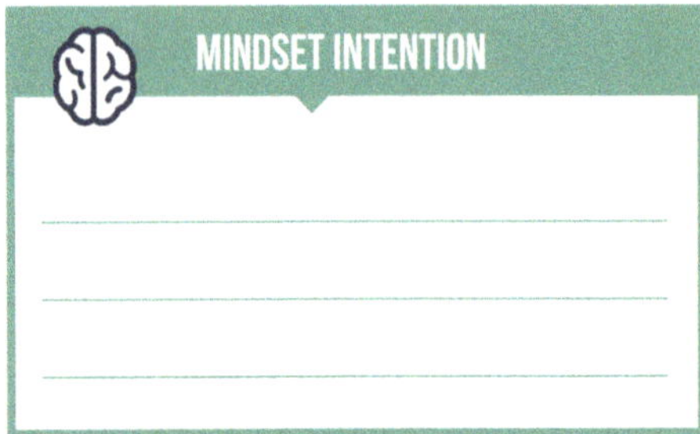

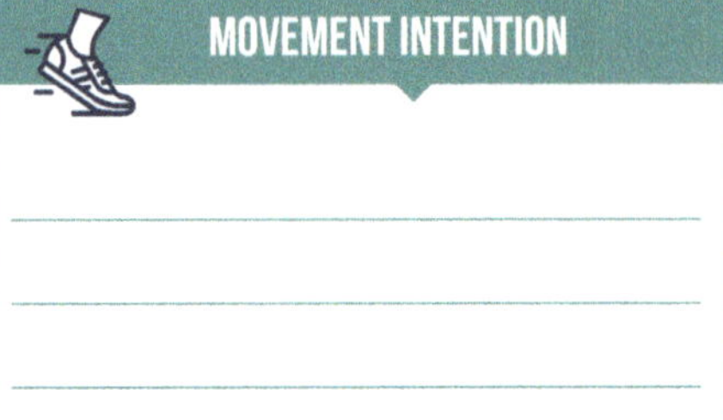

MINDFUL AFFIRMATION:

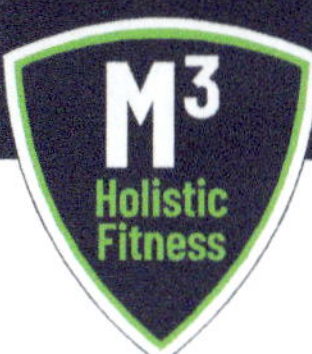

NIGHT CAP

BEDTIME:

HYDRATION   1 2 3 4 5 6 7 8

WHAT DIDN'T WORK TODAY?:

MOVEMENT: ☐

MEALS: ☐ ON ☐ OFF

TODAY'S WINS: 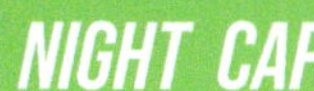

1

2

3

TODAY'S TAKE AWAY:

FOOD FOR THOUGHT FOR THE DAY:

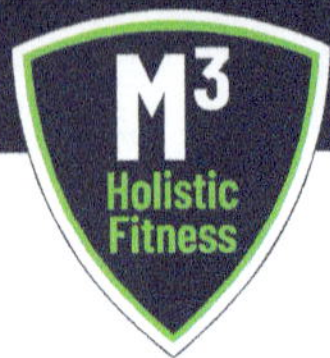

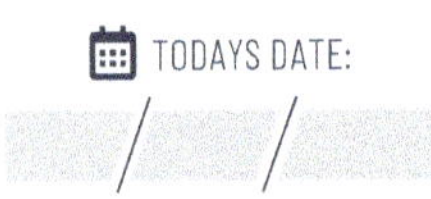

TODAYS DATE: ___ / ___ / ___

ENERGY LEVEL				
MOOD				
BIG ASS GLASS OF WATER				

I AM GRATEFUL FOR:

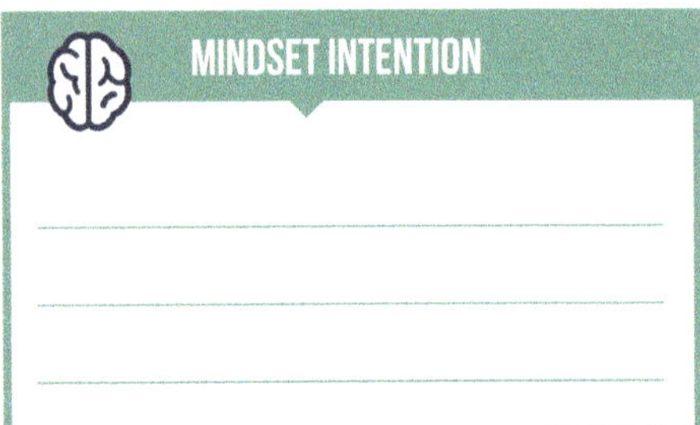

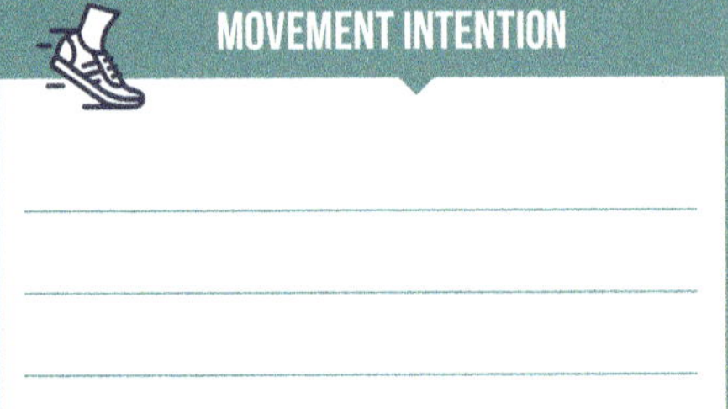

MINDFUL AFFIRMATION:

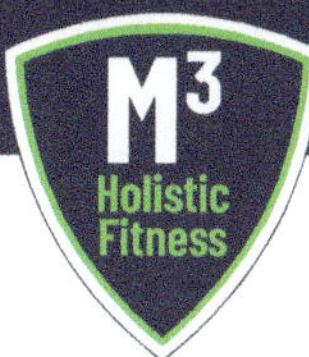

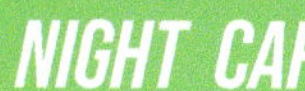

NIGHT CAP

BEDTIME:

HYDRATION | 1 | 2 | 3 | 4 | 5 | 6 | 7 | 8

WHAT DIDN'T WORK TODAY?:

MOVEMENT: ☐

MEALS: ☐ ON ☐ OFF

TODAY'S WINS:

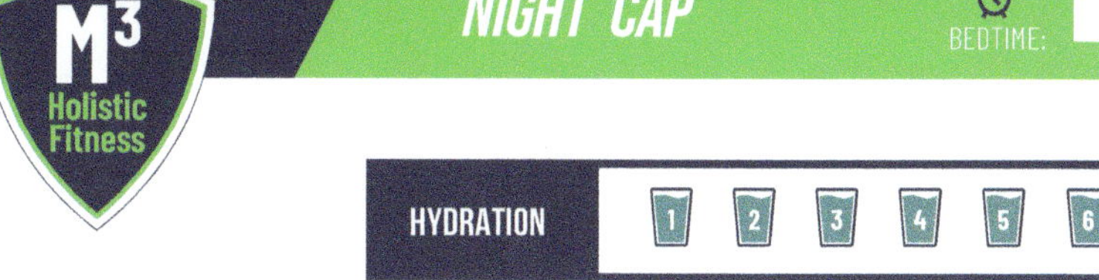

1

2

3

TODAY'S TAKE AWAY:

FOOD FOR THOUGHT FOR THE DAY:

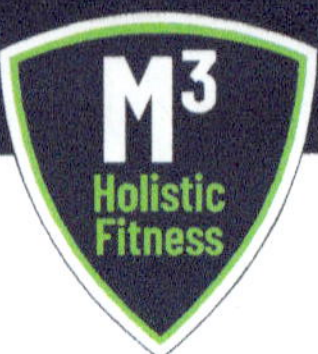

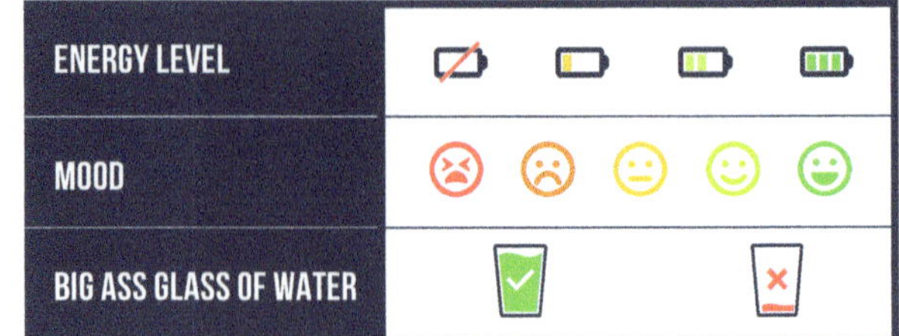

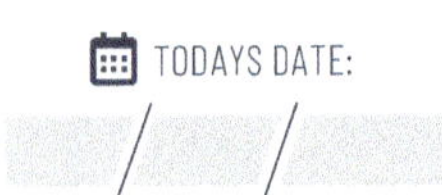

I AM GRATEFUL FOR:

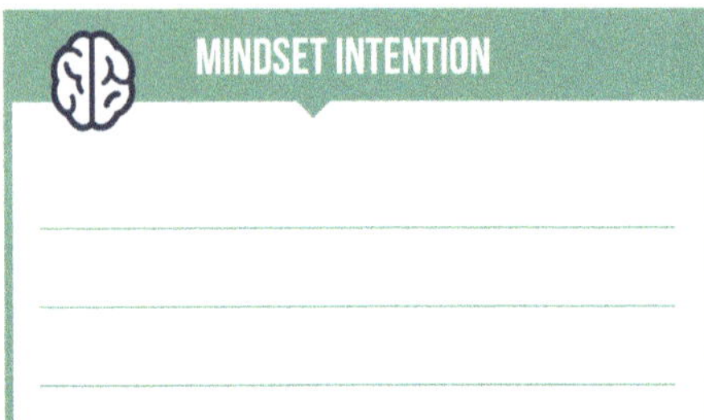

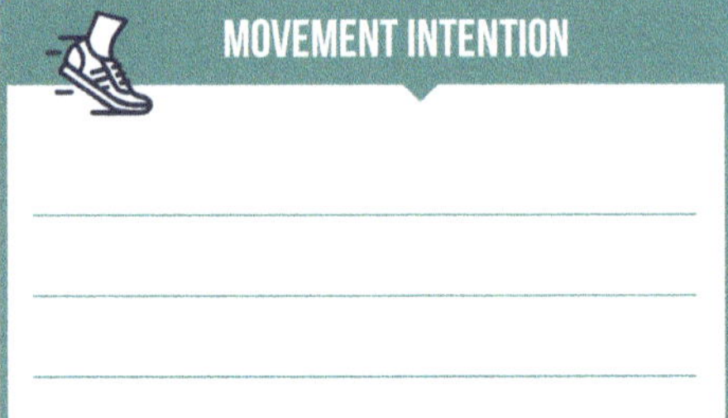

MINDFUL AFFIRMATION:

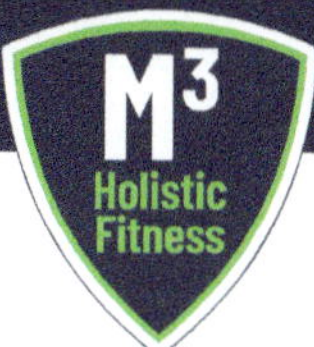

NIGHT CAP

HYDRATION   1   2   3   4   5   6   7   8

WHAT DIDN'T WORK TODAY?:

MOVEMENT:

MEALS: ON OFF

TODAY'S WINS: 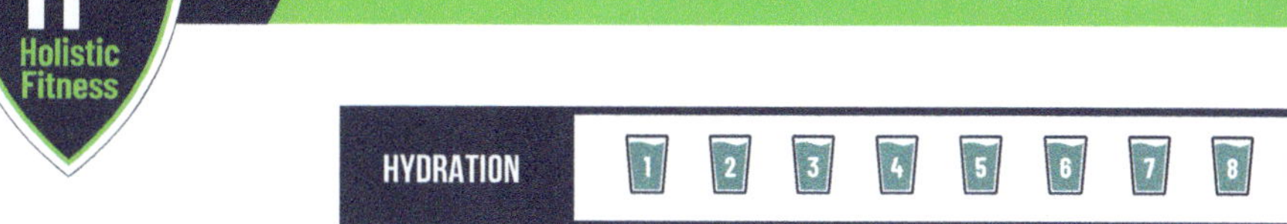

1

2

3

TODAY'S TAKE AWAY:

FOOD FOR THOUGHT FOR THE DAY:

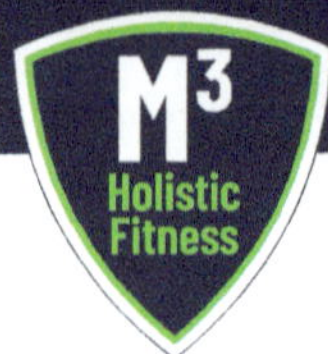

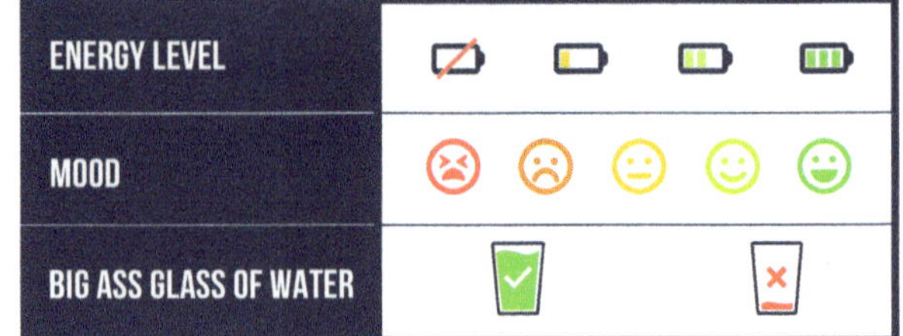

ENERGY LEVEL				
MOOD				
BIG ASS GLASS OF WATER				

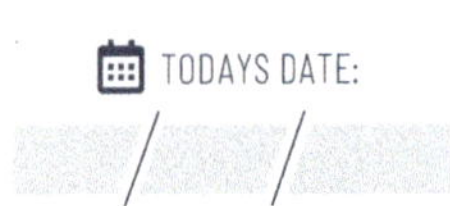

I AM GRATEFUL FOR:

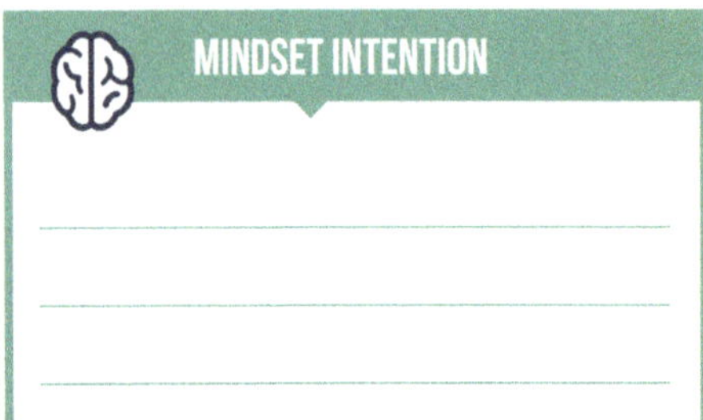

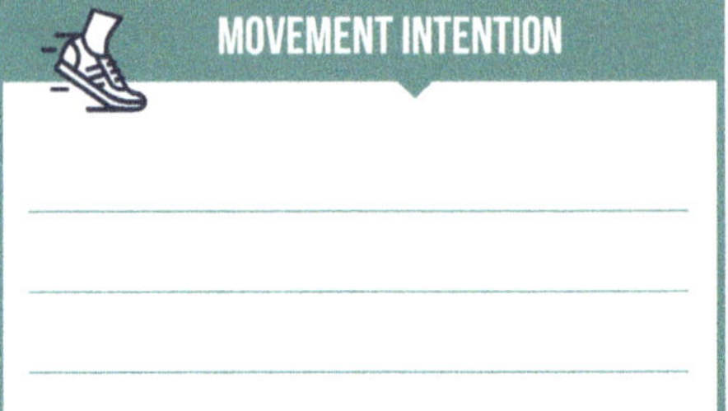

MINDFUL AFFIRMATION:

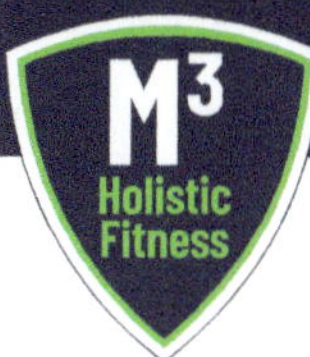

NIGHT CAP

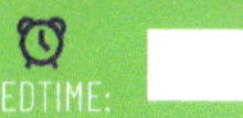

BEDTIME:

HYDRATION 1 2 3 4 5 6 7 8

WHAT DIDN'T WORK TODAY?:

MOVEMENT:

MEALS: ON OFF

TODAY'S WINS:

1

2

3

TODAY'S TAKE AWAY:

FOOD FOR THOUGHT FOR THE DAY:

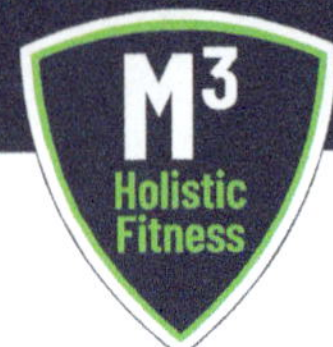

M³
Holistic Fitness

⏰ WAKE UP: ___________   SLEEP: ___ Hrs

📅 TODAYS DATE:

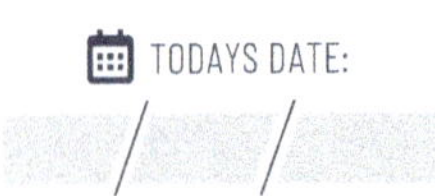

___ / ___ / ___

ENERGY LEVEL	
MOOD	
BIG ASS GLASS OF WATER	

I AM GRATEFUL FOR:

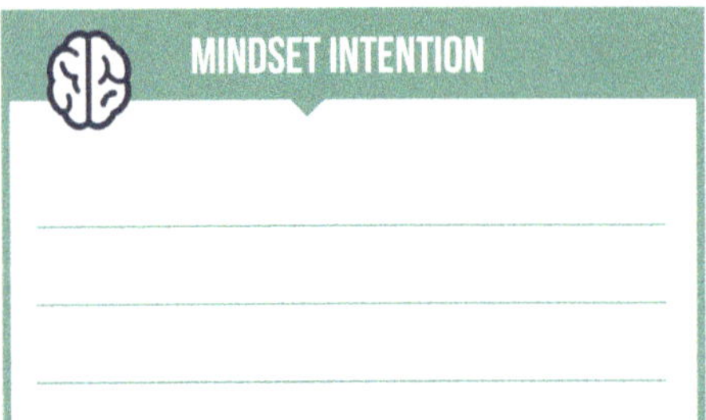

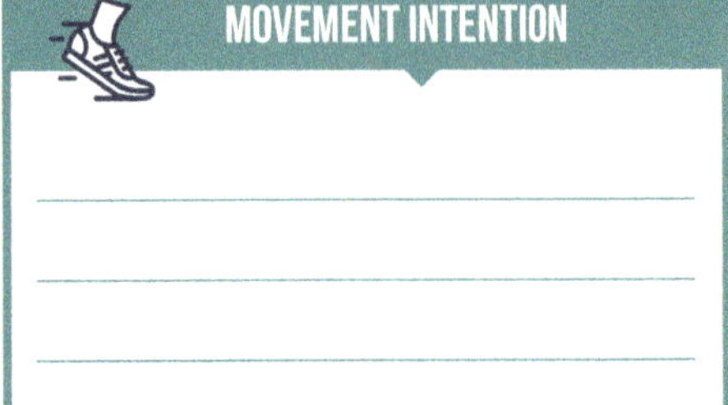

MEALS
INTENTION

MINDFUL AFFIRMATION:

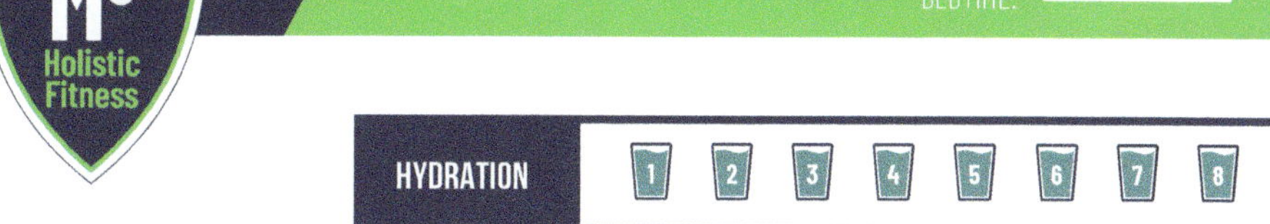

HYDRATION | 1 | 2 | 3 | 4 | 5 | 6 | 7 | 8 |

WHAT DIDN'T WORK TODAY?:

MOVEMENT: ☐

MEALS: ☐ ON ☐ OFF

TODAY'S WINS:

| 1 | 2 | 3 |

TODAY'S TAKE AWAY:

FOOD FOR THOUGHT FOR THE DAY:

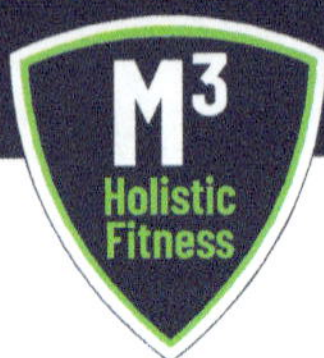
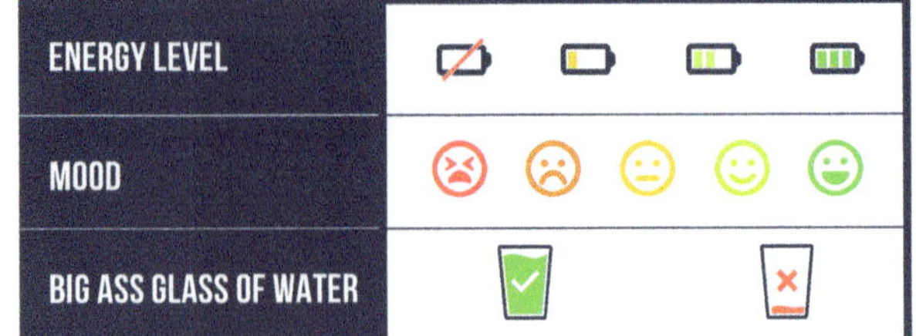

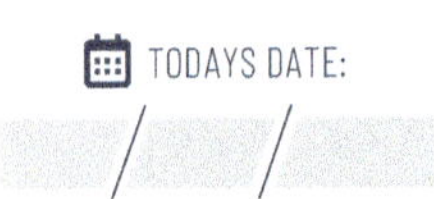

📅 TODAYS DATE:

_____ / _____ / _____

I AM GRATEFUL FOR:

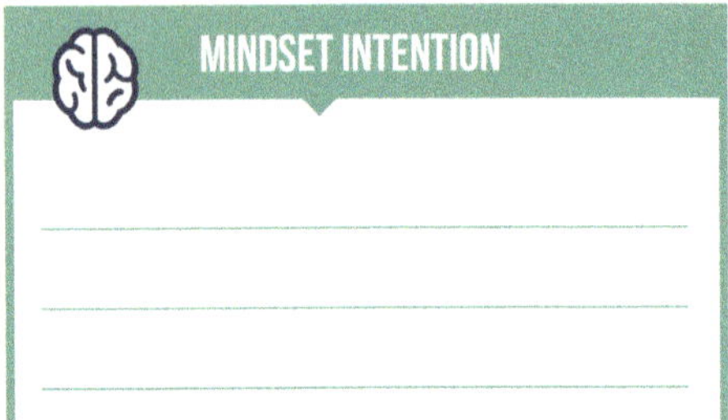

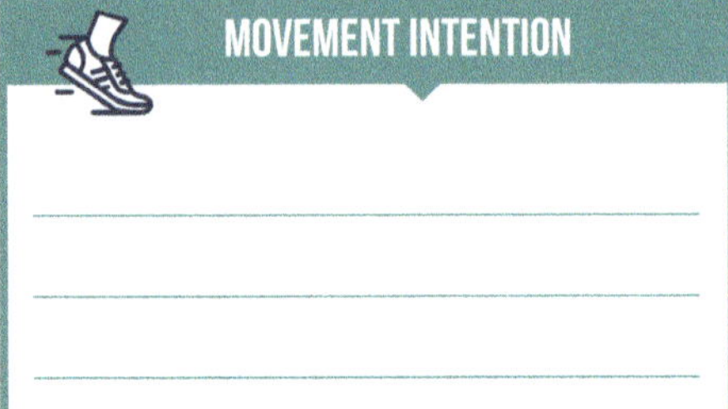

MEALS INTENTION

MINDFUL AFFIRMATION:

HYDRATION 1 2 3 4 5 6 7 8

WHAT DIDN'T WORK TODAY?:

MOVEMENT: ☐

MEALS: ☐ ON ☐ OFF

TODAY'S WINS:

1

2

3

TODAY'S TAKE AWAY:

FOOD FOR THOUGHT FOR THE DAY:

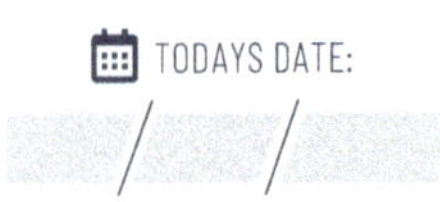

TODAYS DATE: ___/___/___

ENERGY LEVEL	
MOOD	
BIG ASS GLASS OF WATER	

I AM GRATEFUL FOR:

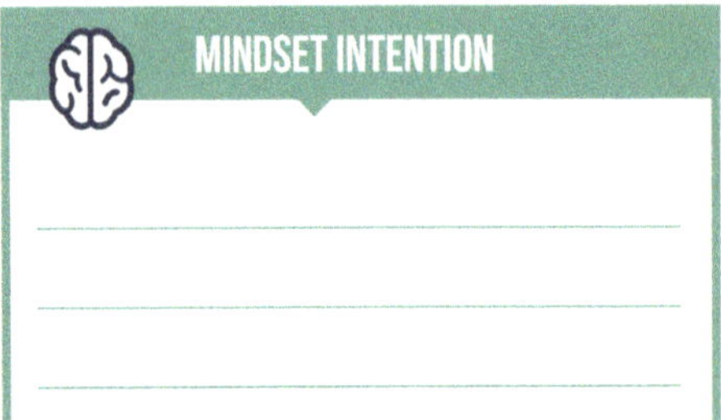

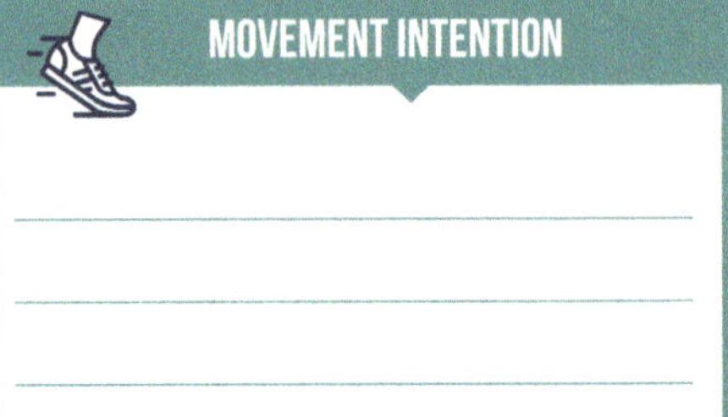

MEALS INTENTION

MINDFUL AFFIRMATION:

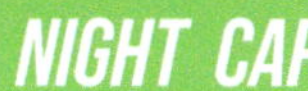

NIGHT CAP

BEDTIME:

HYDRATION   1 2 3 4 5 6 7 8

WHAT DIDN'T WORK TODAY?:

MOVEMENT: ☐

MEALS: ☐ ON ☐ OFF

TODAY'S WINS:

1

2

3

TODAY'S TAKE AWAY:

FOOD FOR THOUGHT FOR THE DAY:

> *The voice in your head that
says you can't do this is a liar.*

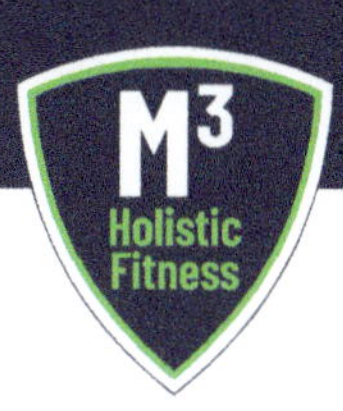

THIS WEEKS WINS:

THIS WEEKS TAKEAWAYS:

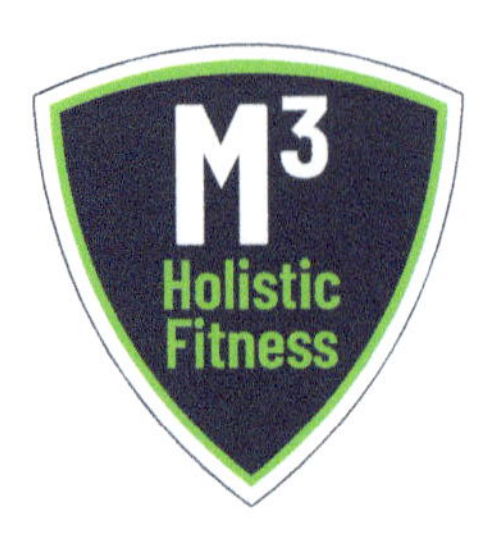

WEEK 12

90-DAY HOLISTIC FITNESS JOURNAL

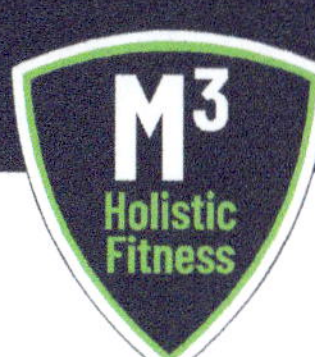

WHAT DOES YOUR LIFE LOOK LIKE?

SATISFACTION

DISSATISFACTION

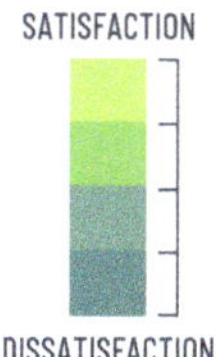

1. Place a dot in each category to indicate your level of satisfaction within each area. A dot at the **center of the circle to indicate dissatisfaction,** or towards the **outer edge to indicate satisfaction.** Most people fall somewhere in between. (see example)

2. Connect the dots to see your M₃ **Circle of Life.**

3. Identify imbalances. Determine where to spend more time and energy to create balance. **This will help you create a better balance for your best Badass Life.**

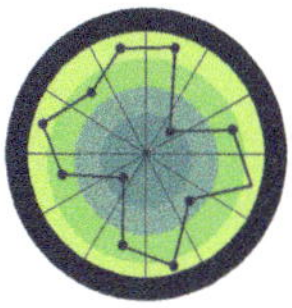

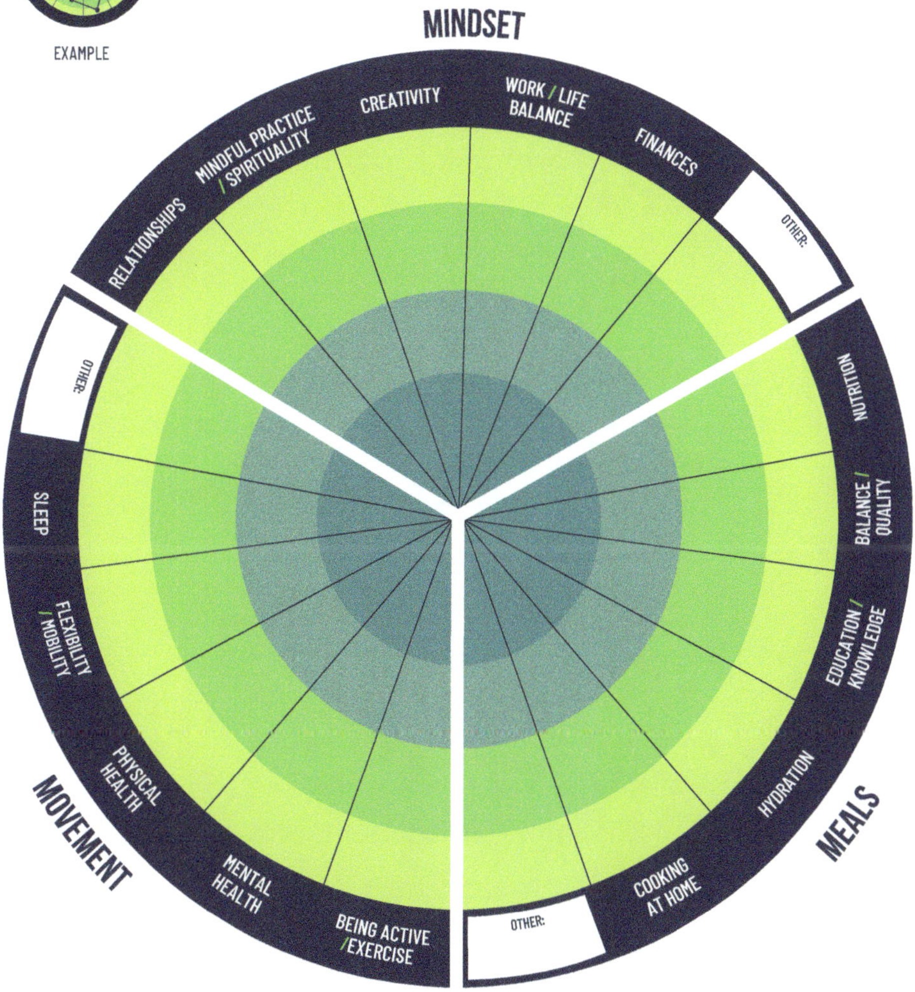

When you change the way you
look at things the things you
look at change.

- Dr Wayne Dyer

M3 Holistic Fitness

MAKE IT HAPPEN THIS WEEK

WEEK OF: ___/___/___

	MINDSET	MOVEMENT	MEALS ON THE PLATE	MEALS OFF THE PLATE
MON				
TUES				
WEDS				
THURS				
FRI				
SAT				
SUN				

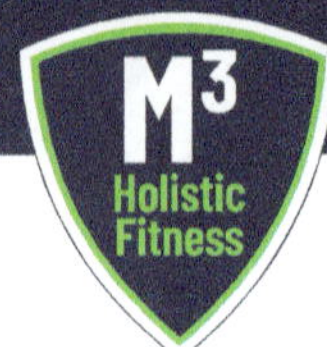

M³
Holistic Fitness

📅 TODAYS DATE: ______ / ______ / ______

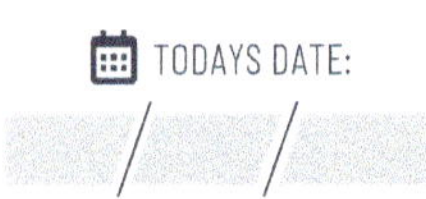

ENERGY LEVEL				
MOOD				
BIG ASS GLASS OF WATER				

I AM GRATEFUL FOR:

____

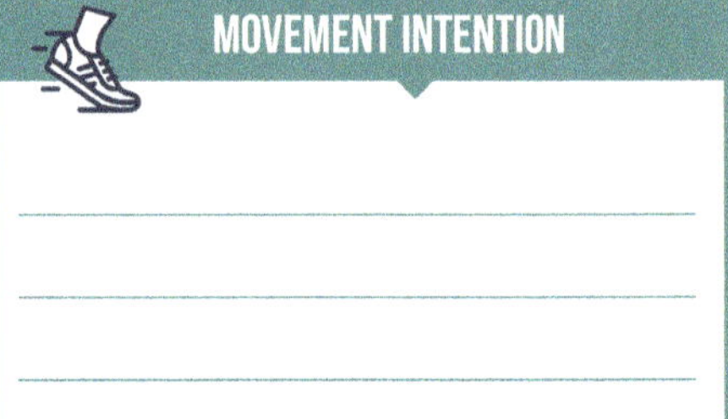

MINDSET INTENTION	MOVEMENT INTENTION

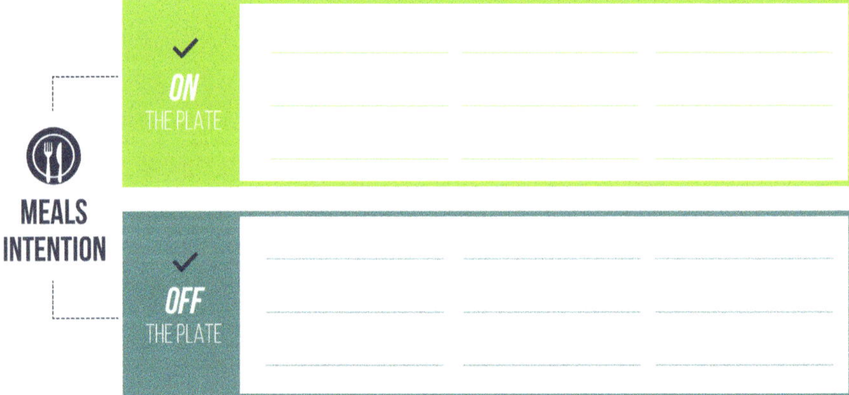

MEALS INTENTION

ON THE PLATE

OFF THE PLATE

MINDFUL AFFIRMATION:

____

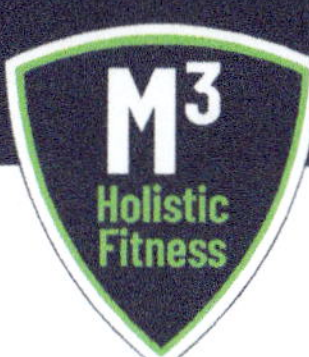

NIGHT CAP

BEDTIME:

HYDRATION 1 2 3 4 5 6 7 8

WHAT DIDN'T WORK TODAY?:

MOVEMENT: ☐   MEALS: ☐ ON ☐ OFF

TODAY'S WINS: 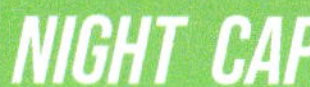

1

2

3

TODAY'S
TAKE AWAY:

FOOD FOR THOUGHT FOR THE DAY:

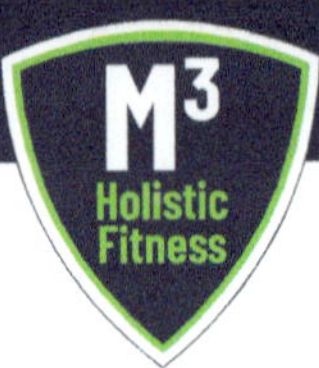

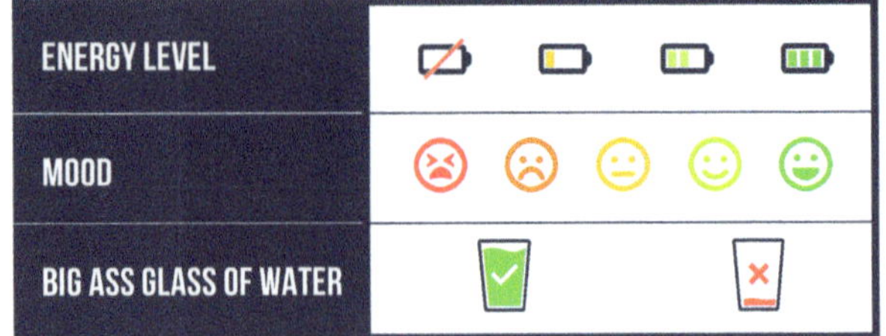

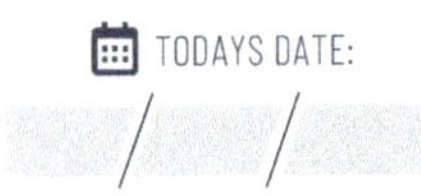

I AM GRATEFUL FOR:

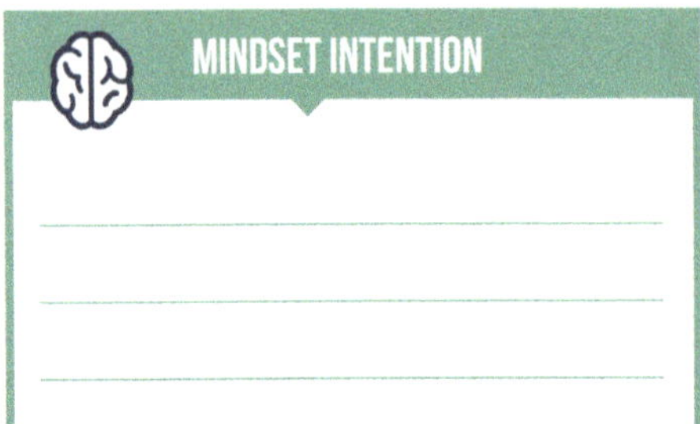

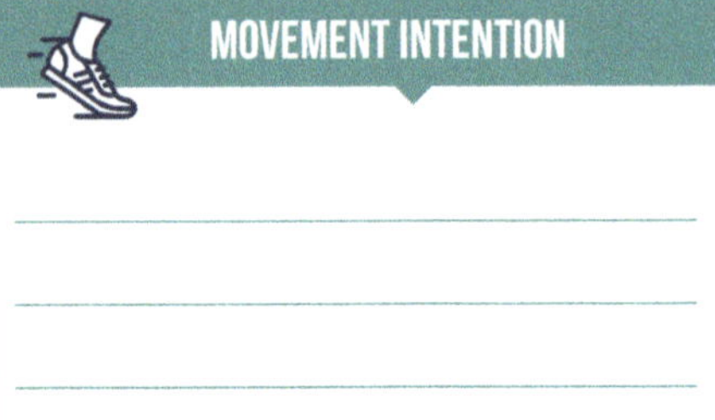

MINDFUL AFFIRMATION:

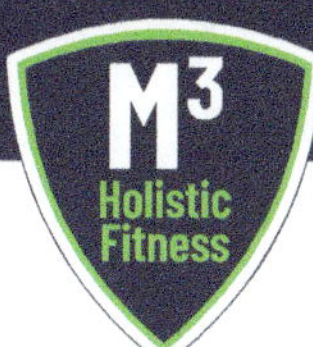

NIGHT CAP

BEDTIME:

HYDRATION   1 2 3 4 5 6 7 8

WHAT DIDN'T WORK TODAY?:

MOVEMENT: ☐

MEALS: ☐ ON ☐ OFF

TODAY'S WINS:

1

2

3

TODAY'S TAKE AWAY:

FOOD FOR THOUGHT FOR THE DAY:

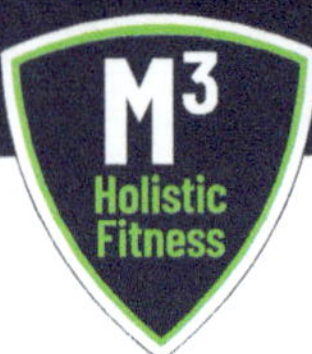

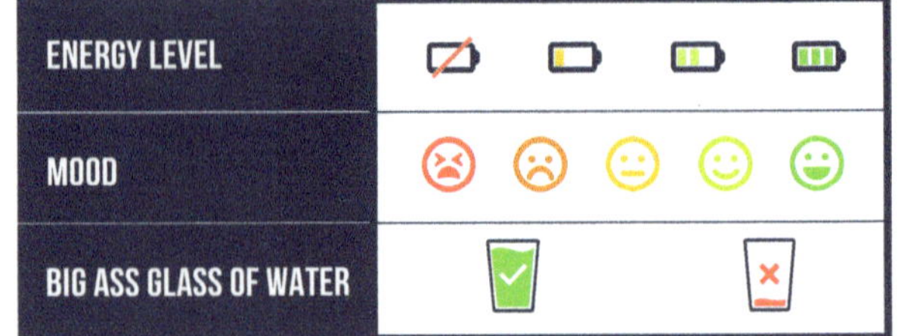

M³
Holistic Fitness

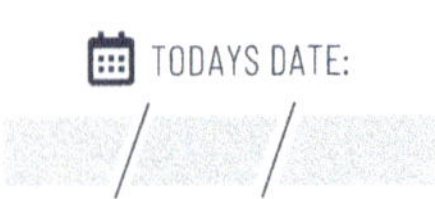
TODAYS DATE: ___ / ___ / ___

ENERGY LEVEL	
MOOD	
BIG ASS GLASS OF WATER	

I AM GRATEFUL FOR:

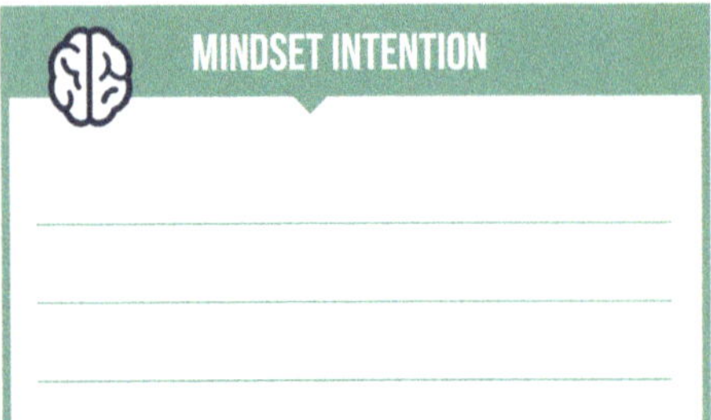

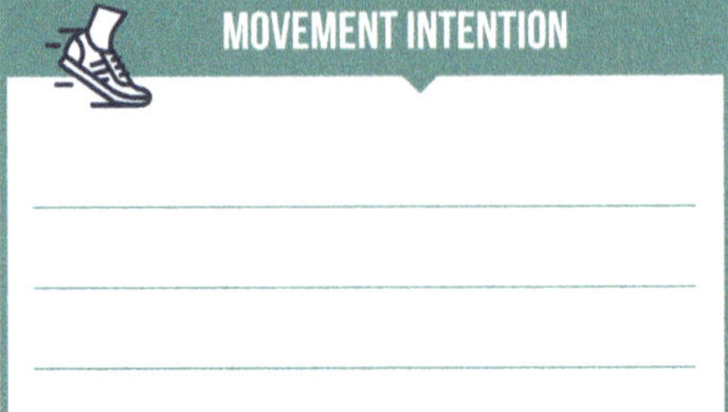

MINDFUL AFFIRMATION:

HYDRATION 1 2 3 4 5 6 7 8

WHAT DIDN'T WORK TODAY?:

MOVEMENT: ☐

MEALS: ☐ ON ☐ OFF

TODAY'S WINS: 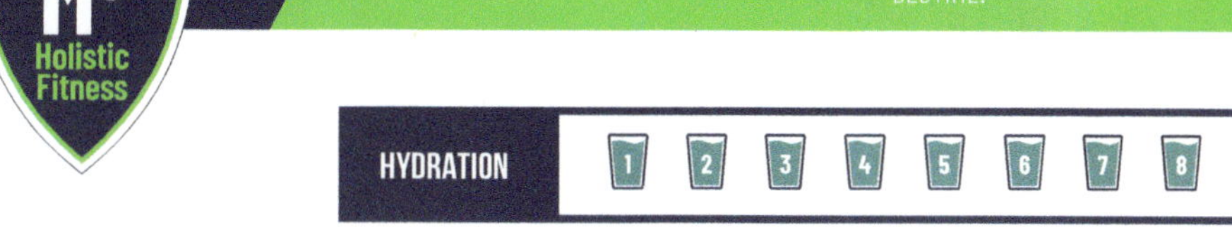

1

2

3

TODAY'S TAKE AWAY:

FOOD FOR THOUGHT FOR THE DAY:

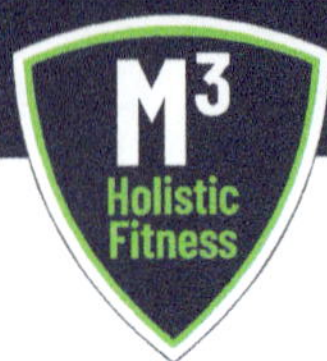

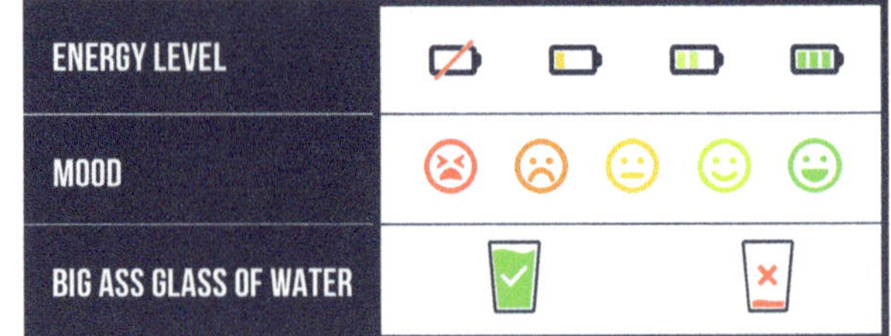

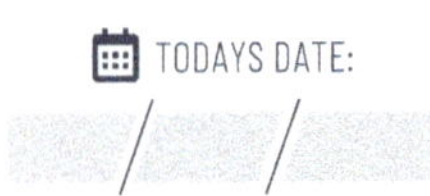

I AM GRATEFUL FOR:

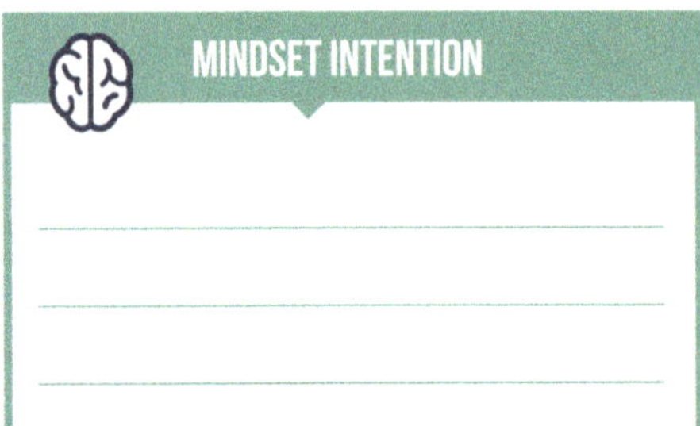

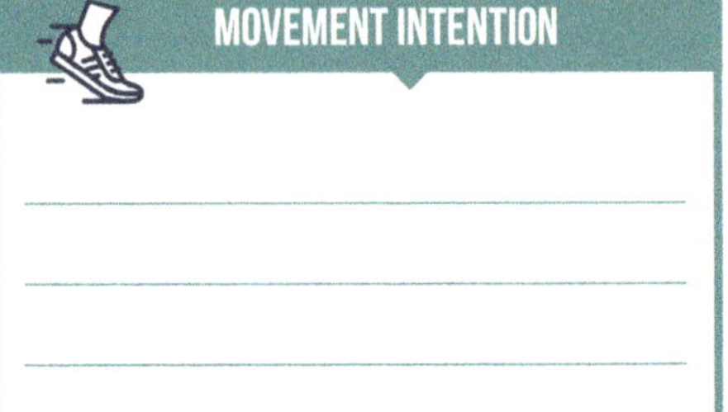

MINDFUL AFFIRMATION:

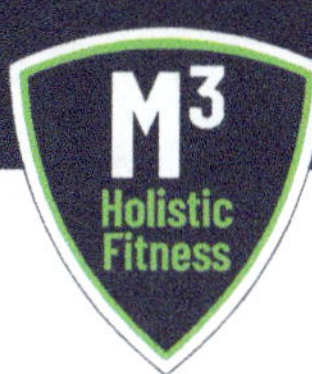

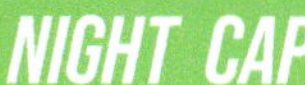

NIGHT CAP

BEDTIME:

HYDRATION   1 2 3 4 5 6 7 8

WHAT DIDN'T WORK TODAY?:

MOVEMENT:

MEALS:
ON   OFF

TODAY'S WINS:

1

2

3

TODAY'S TAKE AWAY:

FOOD FOR THOUGHT FOR THE DAY:

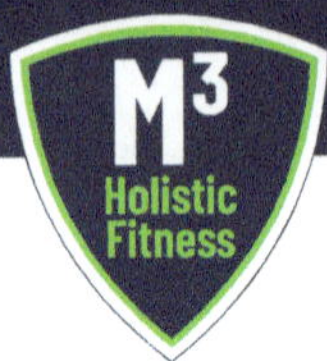

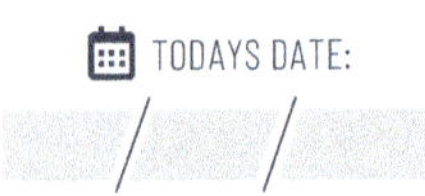

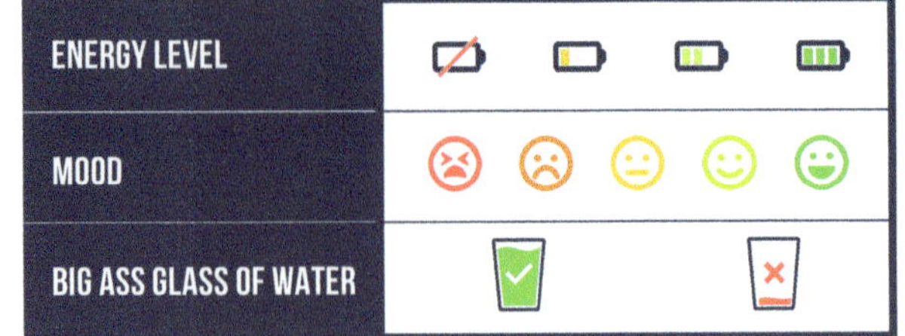

I AM GRATEFUL FOR:

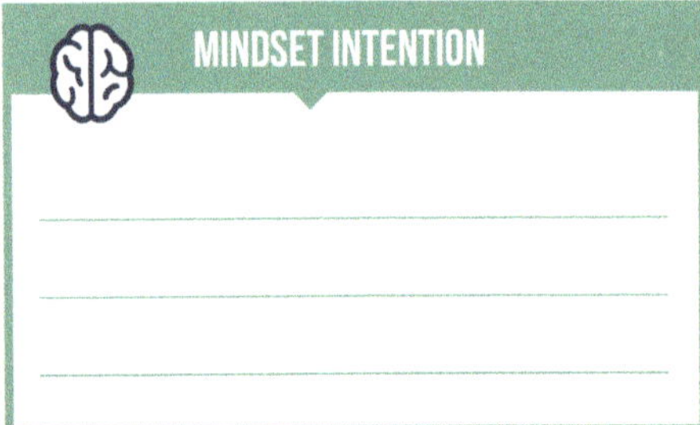

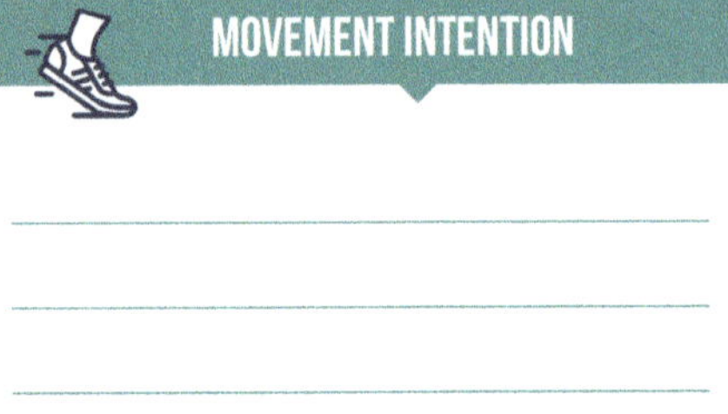

MINDFUL AFFIRMATION:

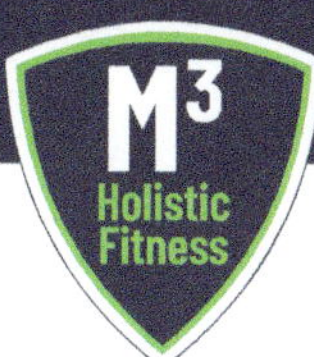

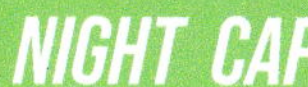

NIGHT CAP

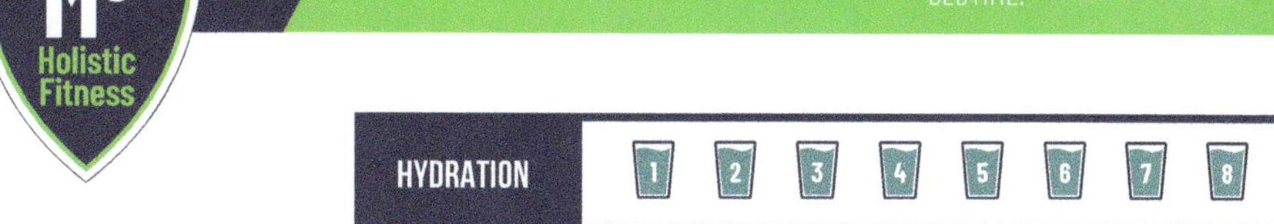

WHAT DIDN'T WORK TODAY?:

MOVEMENT:

MEALS:
ON   OFF

TODAY'S WINS:

1

2

3

TODAY'S TAKE AWAY:

FOOD FOR THOUGHT FOR THE DAY:

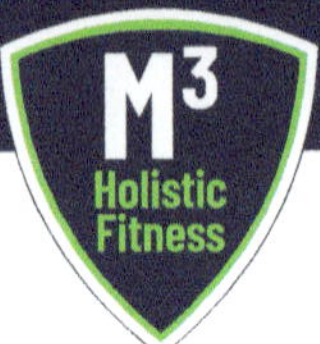

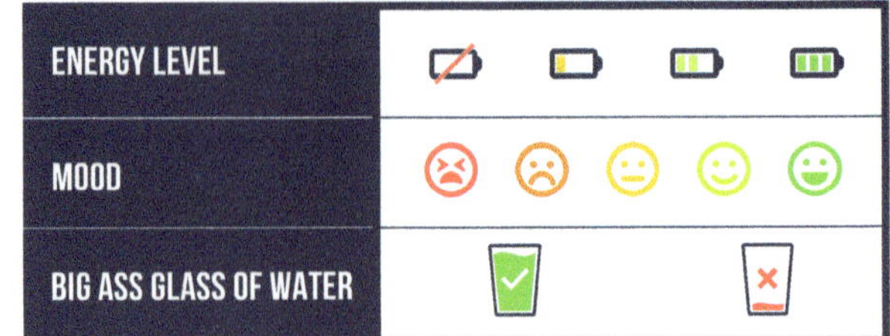

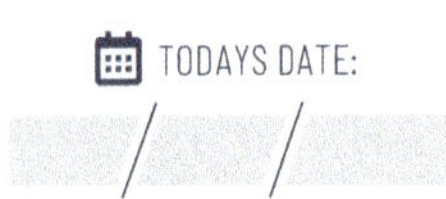

I AM GRATEFUL FOR:

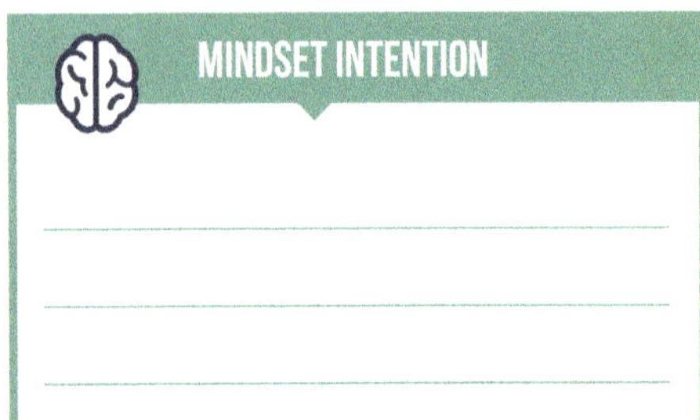

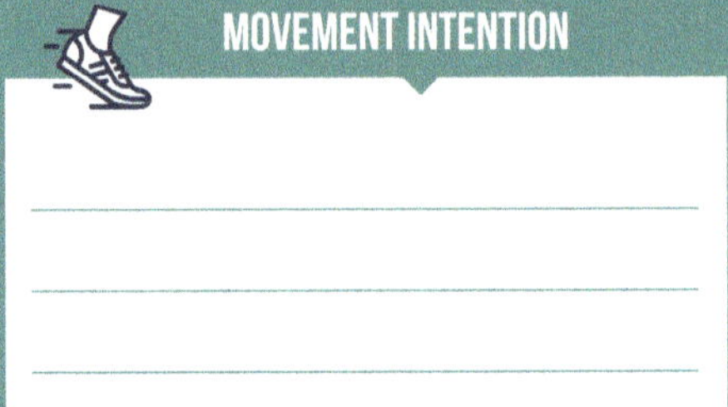

MINDFUL AFFIRMATION:

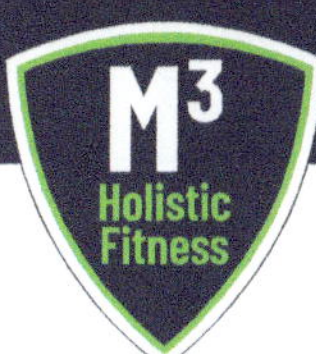

BEDTIME:

HYDRATION | 1 | 2 | 3 | 4 | 5 | 6 | 7 | 8

WHAT DIDN'T WORK TODAY?:

MOVEMENT:

MEALS:

ON   OFF

TODAY'S WINS:

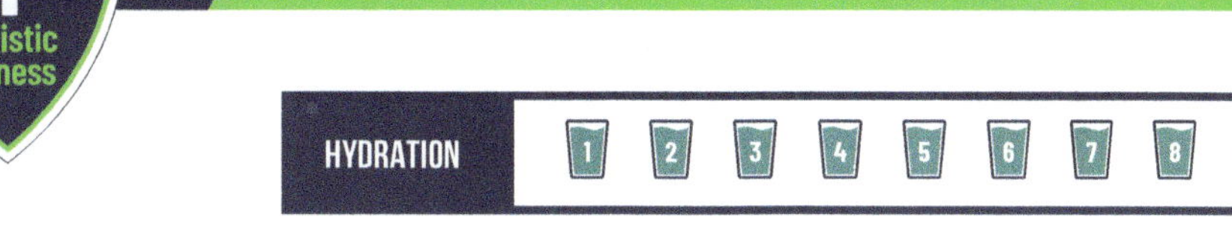

1

2

3

TODAY'S TAKE AWAY:

FOOD FOR THOUGHT FOR THE DAY:

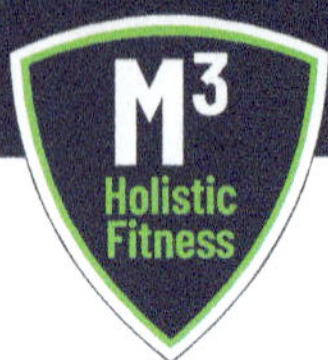

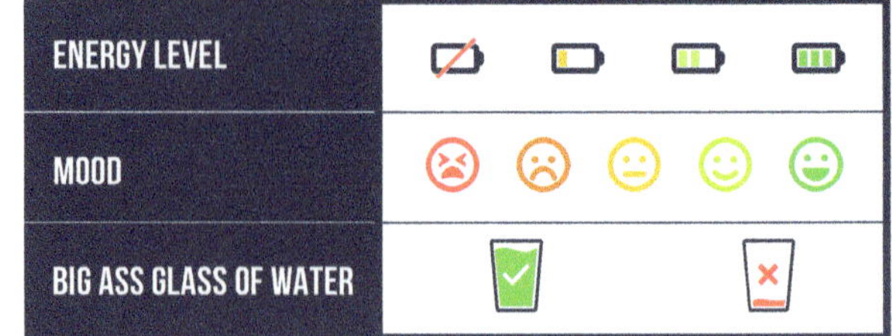

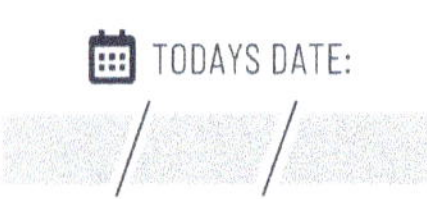

TODAYS DATE: ___/___/___

I AM GRATEFUL FOR:

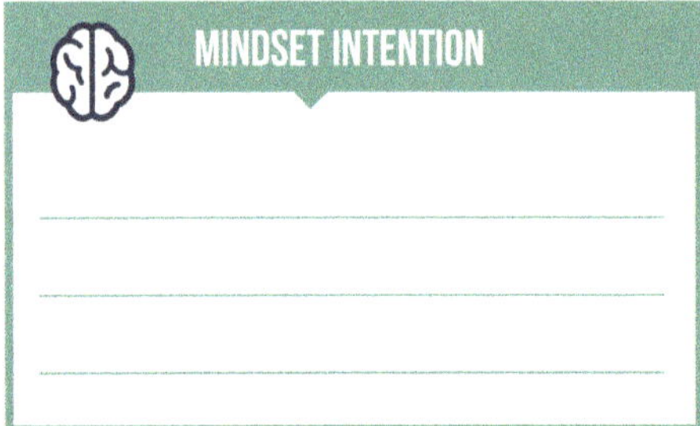

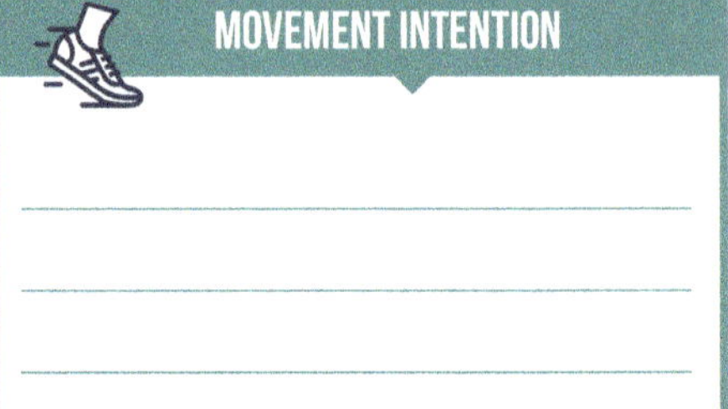

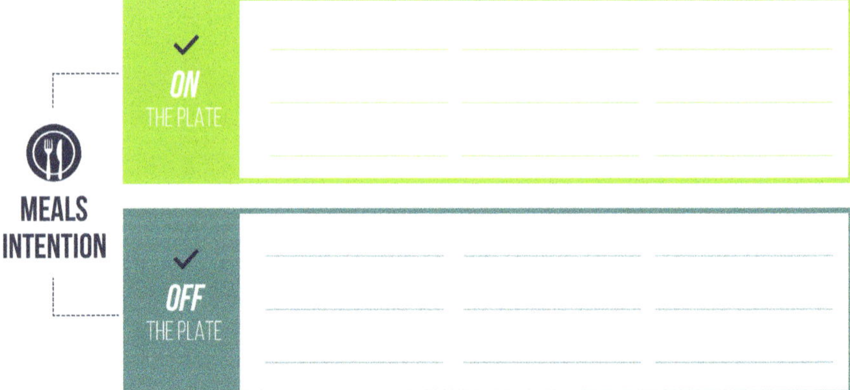

MINDFUL AFFIRMATION:

HYDRATION 1 2 3 4 5 6 7 8

WHAT DIDN'T WORK TODAY?:

MOVEMENT: ☐

MEALS: ☐ ON ☐ OFF

TODAY'S WINS:

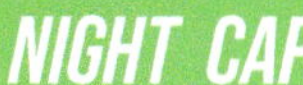

1

2

3

TODAY'S TAKE AWAY:

FOOD FOR THOUGHT FOR THE DAY:

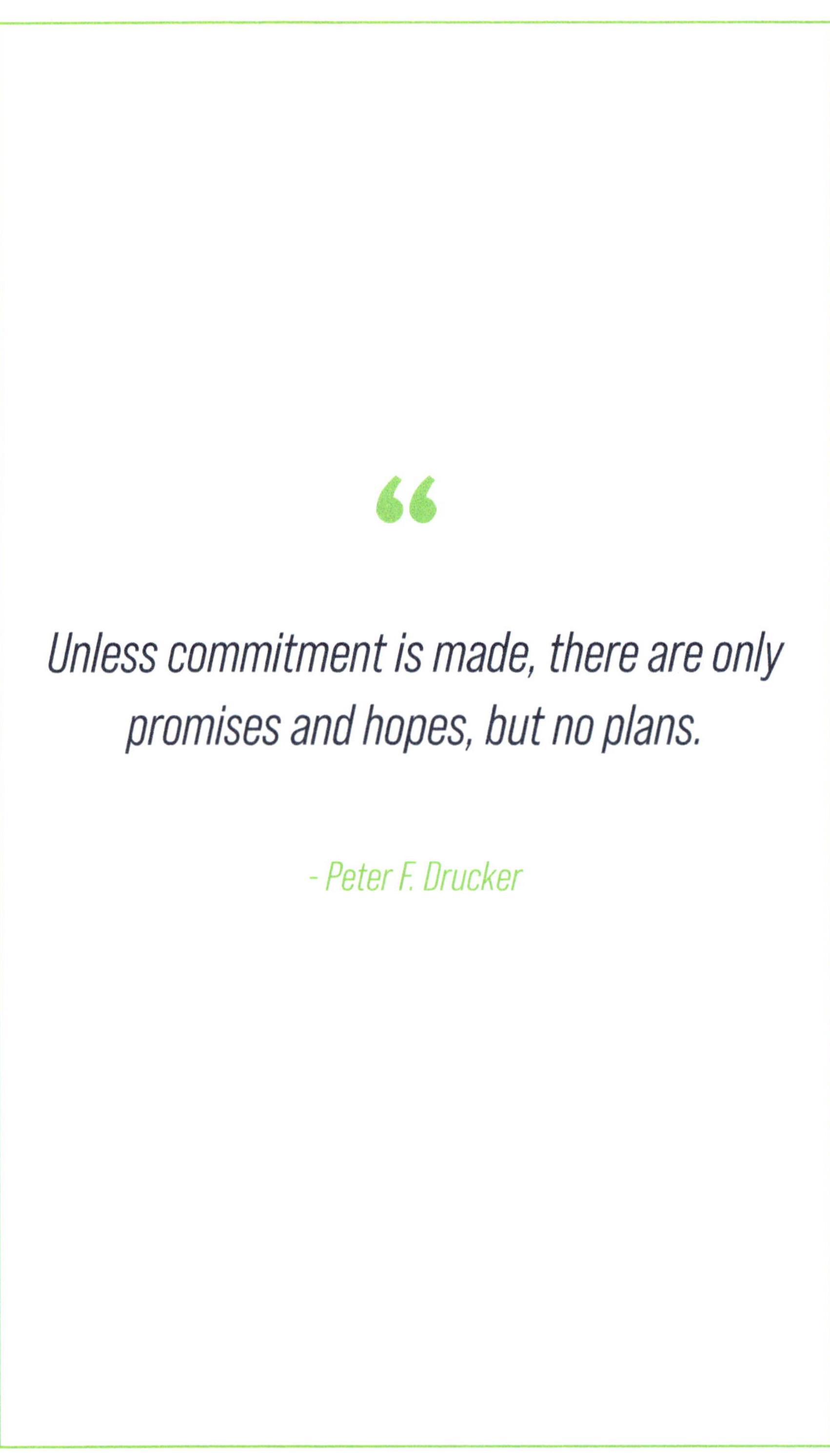

"

Unless commitment is made, there are only promises and hopes, but no plans.

- Peter F. Drucker

Congratulations! Just by making it to this point in the journal,
you've changed your life! You've taken a huge step toward living
your best, badass life. Before you move ahead, I have a question:
Where will you go from here?

THE 90 DAYS IN REVIEW:

What are your top 3 wins from the past 90 days?

What have you learned about yourself additionally these past 30 days?

What is your best next move?
(Start your next 90–Day Rise And Align Journal)

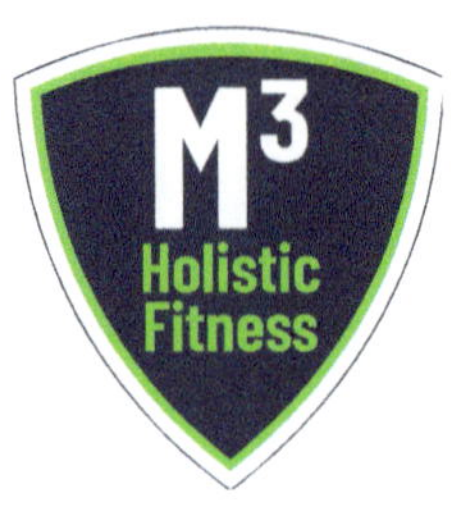

Congratulations!

You have completed your first tour of the 90–Day Rise and Align journal and the M3 Method and now are ready to begin reinventing your life for the road ahead.

As we close the pages of this journey, it's essential to pause and reflect on the transformation that's unfolded and what the future holds for you! This isn't just the end of a journal; it's the beginning of a new chapter in your life, one where holistic health and fitness are not just aspirations but lived realities. You've been equipped with the knowledge and tools to weave wellness into every aspect of your being, creating a tapestry of life rich with vitality, joy, and balance.

Take a moment to celebrate yourself and your journey. Be proud of what you've created, not just in your body, but in your mind and spirit. You've embarked on one of life's greatest adventures the quest for holistic wellness and emerged stronger, wiser, and more vibrant. This is not the end; it's a beautiful beginning. The path ahead is yours to shape, with each step guided by the wisdom and strength you've gained. Here's to you, to your health, and to the incredible journey that lies ahead.

— Dirk

Stay in touch with me at dirkschultz.com